the source

Also by David Cumes, M.D.

Inner Passages Outer Journeys
WILDERNESS, HEALING,
AND THE DISCOVERY OF SELF

The Spirit of Healing
VENTURE INTO THE WILDERNESS TO
REDISCOVER THE HEALING FORCE

Africa in My Bones
A SURGEON'S ODYSSEY INTO THE
SPIRIT WORLD OF AFRICAN HEALING

Mpofu's Grandmother's Loving Lessons:
AND THE WISDOM OF HER WAYS

Messages From The Ancestors:
WISDOM FOR THE WAY

Healing Trees and Plants of the Lowveld

The source
Tshisimane

THE STORY OF AN
INDIGENOUS HEALING CENTER
IN REMOTE SOUTH AFRICA

by David Cumes, M.D.

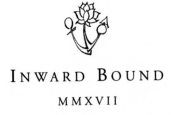

INWARD BOUND
MMXVII

ISBN 978-1-64136-902-2

Printed in the United States of America

First Edition

*Although this book is based on events that
actually happened, and real people, some names
have been changed.*

Dedicated to Maryellen Kelley

It's better to experience the learning
than learn the experience.

WORDS IN A DREAM TO THE AUTHOR

table of contents

I

introduction

We are not asked not to doubt, we are asked to trust.
We are not asked to give what we have not,
we are asked only to give all we have.

We are not asked to embrace all that makes claim on us,
we are asked only to embrace that which ennobles us.
We are not asked to be other than who we are,
we are asked only to become all of who we are.

The Ancestors

THERE ARE SEVERAL REASONS WHY I HAVE WRITTEN THIS book. Firstly, I thought that it was an interesting factual account about a dream I had of the building of an indigenous healing center in one of the more remote regions in South Africa. The exact topography of *"Tshisimane"* (which means the source, a spring, and also the Creator) was revealed to me in a dream; I later located this place in the far north of South Africa. The story explains the many challenges we faced during that time, including land claims that resulted in my eventually leaving the center and moving on. At inception I knew this was going to be a difficult task, but the building of the center was also to take my intuitive understandings to another level. I had always had a dream to have a retreat in the bush in South

Africa, the place of my birth. This story is an account of the actualization of this dream, and the trials and tribulations, as well as the many revelations and rewards, it brought to my life.

Secondly, having been initiated as a *sangoma* in 2002, I was still in the infancy of my indigenous healing practice, and knew that I had a lot to learn. Much of the process of that learning is expressed in this book. Certainly the deepening of my appreciation of African healing wisdom and medicinal plants during my sojourn in the Soutpansberg mountains proved invaluable to me as a traditional healer. The lessons that punctuate the text cannot be found in books, since *sangoma* medicine is an oral tradition handed down over the generations. I also hoped this information would deepen the knowledge of those seeking further enlightenment regarding this ancient, sophisticated form of healing that began in Africa millennia ago. As Paul Simon sings in his song about African music, "These are the roots of rhythm, and the roots of rhythm remain." So, too, are these the roots of healing, and as my *sangoma* mentor confirmed to me, "This original medicine will never change." To this day, when I have concerns about the truth of modern-day complementary or integrative medicine, I return to these roots to see if I can find the same principles at the watering hole of my African "university." If I cannot find it there, I often remain unconvinced about the validity.

The third reason only became apparent much later on during the writing. At the same time that I was in the process of building the center, there was another learning process going on in California that focused around dreams. After my initiation in Swaziland, my friend Maryellen Kelley and I began to receive dreams from a plethora of spirit guides who insinuated themselves into our dreams. Many of these were African and, in addition, Jewish and Celtic mystics began to appear. When

I first wrote the story, because they were not "African," I negligently left them out of the text. It was only when I thought the book was complete that I realized their wisdom was an integral part of my maturation process. I had created a duality where there was none. I could no longer separate the African teachings from the rest. The learning process was just one thing, and all the spirit guides were in collaboration. The ancestors were networking in a much more sophisticated way than I, or even our modern technology, would think feasible. This knowledge is perhaps the most significant for the telling and the reading of this story. It needed to be included, and now it is. These teachings permeated all my experiences, many of which are quoted in the text as this tale unfolds.

I qualified in medicine in Johannesburg, and after completing my internship began a surgical residency. Even during this busy time I had a deep appreciation for the restorative effects of the wild, and I would venture into remote areas with a 4x4 on a regular basis to keep my soul alive while completing five years of rigorous surgical training. In 1975, after becoming board certified in general surgery in South Africa, I emigrated to the United States to begin a urology residency at Stanford Medical Center. In spite of my good fortune in being admitted to Stanford, I still felt something of myself remained lost somewhere in the dust of an African landscape. In 1981, after teaching at Stanford for a year and practicing in Seattle for another, I began a private practice in Santa Barbara, California that I maintain to this day. Santa Barbara felt like home – the ocean, mountains, vegetation and beauty reminded me of my homeland.

the source

You are to give yourself to reconciling the soul's health
with the body's health.

If you do not dare be wholly you, who then ever will?
If you do not lead, whom then can one follow?

There are many forms of transformation, just as
there are many sacred prayers and holy paths.
You are to find the one for you.

Little in my upbringing could have predicted the path I would follow after I moved to Santa Barbara. After a midlife crisis arising from frustration with the direction the medical field was taking and a deteriorating marriage, I embarked on a personal journey that began with an extended visit to the Bushmen of the Kalahari. It was here that I developed an understanding of the power that nature has to induce spiritual transformation, or what I called "wilderness rapture." I wrote a book on this idea titled *Inner Passages, Outer Journeys* (Llewellyn), formed a small company called Inward Bound, and began to take groups of seekers on healing journeys into remote wilderness areas.

While on trips to Peru I was exposed to curanderos or shamans and began to realize they had deep knowledge of healing to which I was not privy, despite all my medical training. When I went back to South Africa, I began to consult the local *sangomas* and *inyangas*. They would answer my queries, but invariably also added, "The bones, they say you should be doing our work. ... The bones say you should be doing African medicine. ... Your grandmother's bone is telling you to be initiated. ... Your ancestors want you back here in Africa!" I had been looking for a meaningful alternative and integrative healing paradigm aside from wilderness healing, but refused to believe that as a left-brained surgeon I was capable of becoming an African shaman. However, after several such readings, all of them given by different *sangomas*, none of whom knew each other, I began to pay attention, although I made no definite plans to proceed. Instead, I wrote a second book called The Spirit of Healing (Llewellyn) that spoke to those ancient principles of healing that much of the medical profession appeared to be ignoring.

Eventually, due to my reluctance, the ancestors revealed themselves directly through a woman *sangoma* who went into trance and became "possessed." She told me in no uncertain terms that I was ignoring my destiny and needed to be trained, or undergo *Thwasa*. She insisted that unless I listened to my ancestors who were "calling" me, my incessant bad headaches (she had no word for migraine), a symptom of the "ancestor sickness," would not go away. At long last I decided to do something about "their" demands, but was still skeptical about my intuitive abilities.

(It is important to note that in the text I use the word "ancestors" in a broad context to include all spirit guides. *Sangomas* are very aware that we all may also have foreign spirit guides that have no relationship to our immediate personal blood line.)

I was drawn to an elderly Zulu *sangoma* in Swaziland who agreed to teach me. P.H. Mntshali, or P.H. as he was affectionately called, began my training on the cusp of the millennium. My third book, Africa in my Bones (New Africa Books), is about the initiation and how profoundly my life has changed and been enriched since that time. P.H. said to me, "You have to tell the Westerners that they have lost the way. They need to know that the cause of many of their problems is neglect of the ancestral spirits. This knowledge will help them get back to what we in Africa know." As my ancestors later informed me:

> *Your mission is to take from there [South Africa]*
> *to bring to here [the United States and the West],*
> *not the other way around!*

It was around that time I met Maryellen Kelley, a prominent educator in Santa Barbara, who began to involve me as a speaker in her adult education programs. Her role in a different form of dream initiation began to take place simultaneously, and will be addressed later in the book.

Various quotes and teachings that enriched what the *sangomas* taught me were channeled to both of us in dreams after the millennium. I have included many of them in this book. A fourth book, compiled by Maryellen and myself, called *Messages from the Ancestors – Wisdom for the Way* (self-published) was released, and some of the sayings from that book are also included here. There are many other profound insights and, where appropriate, they have been added to this text.

In addition to the dreams and the sayings, I also began to get songs in my dreams. Some were chants, some were songs, others were "one liners" with a spiritual message, and some of these also punctuate the text. These songs have been arranged into a series of CDs by myself and a South African musician, Eugene Havenga, and they continue to be downloaded by the spirit world, necessitating yearly visits to Eugene. A fifth book followed, on the messages my African guide, Mpofu, related in dreams, called *Mpofu's Grandmoth-*

er's Loving Lessons (self-published).

The journey that you are about to read chose me, I did not choose it, but I trusted that there was a higher source that knew more than I did. After my initiation, I also began to follow the dream I'd had about this mountainous place somewhere in Limpopo. This book is about literally dreaming the dream, actualizing and living the dream, and then eventually leaving the dream. It also stresses the power made available to us by ancestors or spirit guides who are there to help us if we decide to follow our destiny with trust.

> *Decide what compels you and let all else follow. If you declare your heart, whatever it is, and follow its course, however inexplicable it may seem; all else that you truly want will fall into the flow, but not always as you would arrange it or like it to be or look for it to manifest.*

> *All must be done for its own sake, not for reason of an outcome. All is a journey, not a destination, and it is a continual arriving.*

The *sangoma* walk is one of trust and surrender to something much bigger than oneself. I was later to find out just how true were their words, *"… but not always as you would arrange it or like it to be or look for it to manifest."*

When I look back on my life, I can see that all along the way, and especially since 2000, there were hidden hands that helped guide me. I made many mistakes, and retarded my progress over and over, but eventually was guided or helped myself get back on track. Since the millennium my life has very much been like a treasure hunt in which I follow the clues that

THE SOURCE

come in dreams and as intuitions to the next step in my life path, as directed by a higher source unconfined to the space-time continuum and therefore more all-seeing than myself.

II

initiation
Thwasa

Spirit guides are not subject to time and space
as are we. They are always around,
but not always to be seen; always within call,
but not always to be heard; always present,
but not always to be sensed; always holding us,
but not always to be felt.

A POTENTIAL INITIATE WHO IS "CALLED" BY THE ANCESTORS often becomes ill and will visit a traditional healer for treatment. The *sangoma* will divine and say that he or she is "possessed," and that the only recourse for him or her is to become a *sangoma*. Failure to respond to the ancestors usually is associated with progression of the illness – in my case, incessant migraines. The "ancestor sickness" mysteriously disappears after initiation has begun. The process of being called and then initiated is called "*thwasa*". To become a *sangoma* requires arduous and difficult training. Not just anyone is called and, though sometimes burdensome, the calling is regarded as a gift and a great honor.

One of my first experiences with this traditional healing was at Victoria Falls in Zimbabwe in 1992. I entered the healer's hut and sat on the ground. The *nyanga* threw the bones. I looked, dressed, and talked like a South African, so I was particularly surprised when he correctly told me that I came from a faraway country. He also told me that he saw trouble in my home, big trouble. He said the difficulty was serious and concerned my wife, but he did not see divorce in the bones. Before I had left California for Zimbabwe, my wife and I had separated, and I thought the separation was final. The *nyanga* proved more accurate than I realized since after I returned to California there was a reconciliation that lasted several years. The *nyanga* also told me that I was a doctor and healer, but that in time I would begin to use traditional African methods of healing. My initiation was a testament to his accuracy. The whole experience, though bizarre, seemed intuitively correct at the time.

I was still to hear what other *sangomas* would tell me in future divinations: "You are not listening to your calling. You go here, you go there and everywhere. You search but do not find. You have a gift, a healing gift, a touch gift. There are three ancestors trying to reach you. Your grandmother from your mother's side is the one who will give you the healing power. There is also a youngish uncle, who really loved you. Slowly you will be doing more and more of this kind of work and less regular medicine. There is also the spirit of a black woman close to you. She will assist you in becoming a *sangoma* and throwing the bones. You are already appearing in the bones as if you are a *sangoma*, you just need to complete." Up until this time these messages had not propelled me forward, but after the compelling experience with the *sangoma* who went into trance, I realized I had no other option but to submit. I remained skeptical about the new undertaking and whether, with my cognitive bias, I had any intuitive abilities whatsoever.

*Chant your way across the veil. Spiral into existence spirits
that are needed. There is limitless power from which you
may draw. It will be given to you according
to the measure of your love and trust.*

I had no difficulty embracing this wisdom intellectually, but I had serious doubts as to my abilities to receive the messages from the other side of the veil between worlds. P.H., however, confirmed that the grandmother on my mother's side was the one who would help me become a different kind of healer and that there was a foreign black spirit attached to me who had been a *sangoma* when she was alive. She had been a friend of my maternal grandmother and was the person who would teach me the bones, with his help. The ancestors emphasized that I must become a master of the bones and as good as P.H. himself. At least initially, direct possession was not essential – after all, who would drum for me in America? The bones were going to be my main tool for a new kind of healing.

*There are as many varieties and paths in death as there are in
life. It is not unusual for one to linger between the worlds for a
period of time after death and when called upon may respond
so that the exchange can purify and strengthen both the spirit
of the sentient being and that of the one passing on.*

P.H. was just the mentor I needed to get me started. He was not only the best diviner I was to come across on my journey, but his command of English was impeccable, as was his ability to articulate obscure mystical concepts. He stressed that it was important to be humble. I had received a gift from the ancestors and it was they who would be doing the work. I was only the messenger. My role was to bring this knowledge to the West, where people did not yet appreciate that the source of many problems was a dysfunctional or nonexistent relationship with the ancestors. The ancestor philosophy he was to teach me began in Africa. "Unfortunately, you whites have lost direction, you have taken the wrong road, you are unsupported in life like papers blowing in the wind," he said.

To get more explicit directions from the spirits, P.H. would sometimes enlist the help of a specialist, Mazia, an expert at *Femba*. P.H. Lived near Siteki in the eastern part of Swaziland. Mazia lived thirty kilometers away, close to the Mozambique border. *Femba*, a form of psycho-spiritual cleansing during trance possession, would allow my ancestors to talk to us directly and instruct us exactly how to proceed with the training in the most expeditious way.

Mazia came to P.H.'s homestead the next morning. I was instructed to go to my room. Grass mats were placed on the concrete floor. I sat with my torso bare, my legs outstretched, my arms resting forward between them and my hands open upward on one of the mats. Mazia, dressed in his full *sangoma* regalia, was assisted by his daughter. He chanted and shook a rattle, and very soon a spirit came through him, speaking in English. (Mazia did not know much English.)

Mazia channeled Mpofu, the spirit who would be my guide for divination. Mpofu asked for my white cloth and spat into it, indicating she would be with me wherever I went, especially if I wore the cloth around me. P.H. was visibly pleased and felt confident that he had the right directions on how to proceed with my training. He assured me that Mpofu would make me a master of the bones and umhagate shells. My *Thwasa* had begun.

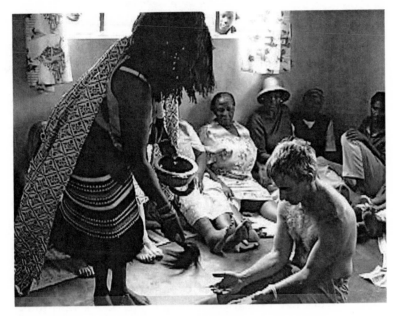

Femba photo

The reading of the bones was quite complex, depending on which were in the front on the mat on which they were thrown, which way they lay, where they pointed, which other bones were nearby, and even sometimes which compass direction they faced. Twice a day, every day, for several hours I sat with P.H. as he interpreted the messages Mpofu gave us through the patterns in which they fell.

P.H. told me that Mpofu, my foreign mandawe spirit, was originally from northern Mozambique near Inhambane and that when her people greeted each other they knelt down and clapped. He added that these people really understood plant medicines.

Miriam, P.H.'s *sangoma* wife, donated the set of umhagate shells from the mangete tree. There were three smaller female ones and three larger male ones. P.H. and Mazia showed me how to throw and interpret them. These confirmed or disputed and added further emphasis to the reading.

Ancestors do not abide arrogant people. Much of a *Thwasa*'s training is to practice humility, which is implicit in the indigenous healing tradition and pervades its rituals. Before entering the *ndumba* (healing hut), the *sangoma*, the attendants, and the client remove their shoes, bow, and once inside, they kneel, clap twice and perform other acts that demonstrate respect and reverence for the ancestors.

Every morning and evening I underwent purification by steaming. A fire was lit under a large three-legged cast iron pot. P.H. added special purifying medicinal herbs, or *muti*. Once the pot had boiled I would sit down on a small wooden stool with the steaming pot between my knees. A blanket thrown over my head covered me completely so that none of the medicated steam was lost. After about 30 minutes of profuse sweating I would emerge energized from the steaming aromatic *muti*. It was mid-summer in Swaziland, and the temperature and humidity were already extremely high, conditions that contributed to effective cleansing. P.H. would brush and "cleanse" me with his buffalo-tail whisk and make incantations to bring my ancestors close by. After the steaming I would pour the contents of the pot into a plastic basin, add some cold water, and wash my entire body with the medicated water. As the day cooled down and the sun began to set, it was a magical time. Still, I had serious doubts as to whether this process would really mature for me. I would acknowledge the ancestors as I faced all four directions. The rest of the day I spent trying to learn Siswati, the Swazi language, which is similar to Zulu. I talked to

P.H.'s children, meditated, walked and did yoga.

After a few days of purification, P.H. brought me a black clay pot filled nearly to the top with water and special *muti*. I was instructed to beat the solution with a stick so that it foamed up. I would take some foam on my finger and place it on my forehead, my heart, and between my shoulders. After that I would slurp up the bubbles by putting my mouth into the mouth of the pot. Finally I washed my face with the foam. This ritual occurred twice a day while kneeling down on a goat skin mat. In the morning I would face east and in the evening, west. The foam was special food for the ancestors and would bring them close to me. I also prayed to them and made requests concerning my journey to become a new type of healer. The brew, called budlu, was a recipe of different herbs that would magically foam out over the edge of the pot as it was beaten with a stick. The ancestral cappuccino tasted quite pleasant, but did have a limited shelf life. There was no refrigeration and even though it was covered and placed in a cool spot, it had to be replenished every few weeks. As one of my friends in California later said to me, "Oh, a twice daily 'foam call' to the spirits."

P.H. told me that, before I left, sacrifices would be necessary to complete my connection to the ancestors. He and Mazia had agreed that the goat sacrifice should be left for a later date. They were concerned that all the spirits, good and bad, would be attracted by such an offering and that this might bring unwanted intruders. They settled on a chicken only for this early stage of the training. Miriam and I drove off to the market in Siteki and bought a white hen.

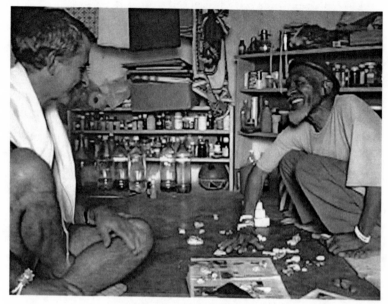

P.H. teaching me the bones

After three weeks, P.H. was satisfied with my initial grasp of the bones and this phase of my training seemed complete. I was to return at a later date for a goat sacrifice. The bone gleaned from this would be crucial for the completion of my collection. P.H. stressed that each teacher's method of divining was unique and depended on the custom of the individual spirit presiding. I now needed to develop confidence with what I had learned and slowly deepen my connection and intuitive understanding with Mpofu.

Before I could leave, there was one thing left to do. This was performed in the *ndumba* or healing hut, with me seated on a stool gazing out the door to the east. The ancestors were greeted and an incision made on the crown of my head. I was surprised that I had no misgivings about this surgical procedure but was gratified all the same that the shaving blade he used was a new one. *muti* was pressed into the incision to complete the bonding to the ancestors. The incision was the port through which they would enter during possession, in dreams, or when I threw the bones. The incision would also enable the ancestors to travel with me back to California and wherever I went. P.H. warned that I was carrying them, and therefore my behavior must be impeccable. When I returned home I was to set aside a special area in the house dedicated to them. There I could perform my rituals and throw the bones until such time that I could house them in their own *ndumba.*

He also gave me the *mutis* I would need in California with detailed instructions. There were herbs for purifying my home, office, and the *ndumba* I was to build. There was *muti* with which to make foam, a plant for purification after sex, and powder to empower any new bones acquired in Johannesburg. This powder could also be taken orally to assist in reading the bones. There were other instructions with regard to food offerings, how to talk to the ancestors, rules with regard to sex and concerning menstruation, how to behave in the *ndumba* and so on. There had to be a special plate for Mpofu, and I must charge a small fee for all consultations. A small token of this fee was to be placed in Mpofu's plate as a sign of thanks to her. He reminded me that a few bones I still needed were missing, and that I might be able to get them in Johannesburg.

The initial part of the training was complete. I said goodbye, told them I would be back in April, and took the road south through the border gate at Golela. As I drove into South Africa, I could feel the whole top of my head tingling. The ancestors are with me, I thought. I also noted that the persistent pain that I'd had in my right shoulder had disappeared.

After I arrived in Johannesburg, I went to the *sangoma* market where I completed my inventory of bones. These included wild pig, or *Ingwelubi*; lion, or *Bubesi*; *Mfeni*, the baboon bone; *Sambane*, the anteater; and *Impisi*, the hyena. The hyena bone, the thief that comes in the night, was essential for locating a lost or stolen object. Just before leaving the Mai Mai market, and the *sangoma* woman who attended the small stall, I asked, "Do you have any bags?" I still lacked a bag to hold the bones. She pointed above her head where at least a dozen attractive skin bags hung from the rafters of the ceiling. Immediately my eye caught one that was distinct from the rest. I asked, "What is that one?" She said with a lilt in her voice, "*Yebo*, that one is *Mpofu*." I was astonished and bought the *Mpofu* bag for Mpofu. I left the next day for California with Mpofu, all my ancestors, my bones in the bag, a grass mat, and my *muti*. When I returned to Santa Barbara and told a friend about all the extraordinary events, he mused, "Did you declare your ancestors when you went through customs?"

I began throwing the bones for some of my friends and acquaintances and, once I became a little more confident, for a few others as well. P.H. had told me that I must charge for the readings, and at the beginning I charged one dollar. In *sangoma* tradition an exchange of energy, usually in the form of money, is always required for a reading, to thank the ancestors and provide for the *sangoma*.

Many of my early clients were familiar with other divining methods such as Tarot cards and the I Ching, and were intrigued by the whole idea. The bones, however, seemed to go beyond these techniques. They spoke to the cosmology of the human condition no matter what the culture. They revealed information concerning one's home, money, spouse or significant other, ancestral and foreign spirits, travel, the shadows over one's life, what it is the heart yearns for, one's destiny, etc. – any topic at all. People's interest was piqued, not just because the readings were accurate, but because of the mystique and the ancient African origins of this diagnosis.

Due to my circumstances, P.H. gave me permission to come and go for a month at a time for the training so that I could also nourish my medical practice in Santa Barbara. This happened two or three times a year over a period of two years.

In April of 2000 I returned for the second time. Almost immediately after I arrived, P.H. checked in with the bones and the ancestors. He was pleased to hear I had been practicing successfully in California and that friends, acquaintances, and others were appreciative. P.H. advised me that a goat had already been obtained to sacrifice to the ancestors, but that we again needed to see Mazia and get explicit instructions from the ancestors. We checked in with Mazia who, in addition to other instructions, said that we would need to not only sacrifice a goat, but a chicken as well.

Someone woke me one morning at 5 a.m. "P.H. wants to test you," he said as he ushered me into the *ndumba*. I sat on the floor while P.H. looked at me with a faint smile.

"I want to know if you remember what you have been taught: are the bones talking, are you aligned with your mandawe teacher, has your practice developed?" I didn't answer, as I was quite intimidated at being tested.

"Now tell me about the goat we have found for you. Is it white or black?" he said.

I threw the bones. "It is white."

"Is it male or female?"

A second throw. "It is a female"

"Where is it?"

"It is behind me and to the right," I said.

P.H. was visibly pleased. His diligent mentoring had not been for nothing.

"Is it inside or outside the *kraal* (a cattle enclosure)?"

"Inside." I hesitated, misreading the metaphor.

He corrected me, "It is outside, can't you see?" I surprised myself that all the other answers had been correct and could not fathom how I was getting all this highly specific information from the bones.

On another morning I was dragged sleepily into his hut again, but this time to throw bones for Mazia. Mazia was a powerful *sangoma* and I was even more uncomfortable and apprehensive having to divine for him. P.H. picked up on my reluctance and said, "Do not apologize for yourself, just read it!" I did, and was again surprised at my accuracy in interpreting the display that Mpofu had so masterfully manipulated with her energetic powers.

The daily purifications and foam drinking continued as before. P.H. had now constructed a mini-sweat lodge, big enough for only one person. It looked like a tiny Bushman hut, but instead of grass for walls there was plastic sheeting and one or two blankets thrown over the top. The familiar three-legged pot with water and *muti* inside was placed in a depression in the center of the floor of the hut. Red-hot rocks from a fire outside were dropped into the pot with a spade by one of P.H.'s sons in attendance. The plastic was drawn over the tiny door as the solution bubbled and boiled and the sweating began. Periodically, as the steam dwindled, more rocks were deposited in the pot. A cup of water was on hand, and a small amount of cold water could be added to the pot to stop it from boiling over and to prevent serious burns. I sat on a brick with my legs astride the pot and tolerated the intense cleansing, which lasted 35 or 40 minutes.

I also spent time reading and thinking, among other things, how it would feel to be possessed, to be so ego-free that my persona could step aside and allow another entity to take over. When I questioned P.H. about this, he did not think I would have any trouble at all. P.H. assured me that, at least at this stage, it was not necessary for me to be possessed, that I could get the same information from the bones. He would often say to me, "The bones are the big boss!"

The next day P.H. pulled me into the *ndumba*. We rehearsed what I had to say when the goat and chicken were sacrificed to the spirits: "I offer the goat to you to honor you all together on my behalf, to do my work with a full heart and full clarity, and to strengthen my practice and remove all obstacles. I thank you for my gift and confirm my commitment to my calling."

We went outside to where the white goat was tethered to an acacia tree. P.H. told me that white goats were hard to come by and that we were lucky to have one. Ndoda, his son, grabbed the rope around the goat's neck and I held onto the horns. Together we pulled the four-legged into the *ndumba*. I said my prayers to my grandfathers and grandmothers.

The next time I saw it was on my return from shopping with Miriam. It was suspended from a tree branch, skinned and lifeless. P.H. was busy butchering it when I walked over. He removed the throat and the surrounding strap muscles and gave them to Ndoda to *braai*, or barbecue.

"This part of the meat is important for you to eat, since now you have found your *sangoma* voice," P.H. said to me.

Several days later I entered the *ndumba* where I found the

white chicken lying docilely on the floor, its legs immobilized with string. Kneeling at the altar in the *ndumba*, I repeated the same invocation to the ancestors, but this time the offering was the fowl. Ndoda brought in a basin of water and I was given three different types of *muti* to sprinkle in the water. Mazia showed me how to use the foot of the chicken to scatter the *muti*, which was placed in a plastic lid on top of the chicken's claw. As each ingredient was added Mazia stirred the water with the claw, first the left, followed by the right.

Mazia opened the chicken's mouth and incised the corners until blood dripped into the water. A few feathers were added to the offering. The chicken was completely passive during the ritual and never cried out or struggled. Ndoda took the two-legged away to be slaughtered while I found a place to strip and bathe myself fully in the sacred blood-colored solution. When I returned to the *ndumba*, P.H. removed a chicken feather from my hair.

On my return home I would frequently get concerned questions about this seemingly barbaric practice. I would always stress the sacredness of the ritual and that the meat was always eaten, enjoyed and shared with the ancestors. If anything it was more personal and real than buying meat already packaged in the supermarket where one had no connection, spiritual or otherwise, with the animal.

I was immersed in ritual. My stomach and intestines had been foam cleansed, my skin sweated, and my body purified. The party for the ancestors now began, and we all sat in the *ndumba* and enjoyed the celebration of *braaied* (barbecued) goat and chicken meat, wine, and sorghum beer. The home-made traditional beer had a subtle delicate taste, better than that of the wine from the Cape. A small amount of meat, wine, and beer was offered to Mpofu and to each of the grandmothers and grandfathers respectively and respectfully. I felt quite emotional and very content, and I realized that this ritual had a more powerful effect on my soul than my intellect had been willing to concede. I expressed my profound gratitude to P.H. and Mazia. Mazia busied himself with one of the bones from the goat, cleaning it and boring a hole down the center so I could wear it as a bracelet. I took up the other bone and cleaned off the ligaments, tendon attachments, and cartilage. This bone also needed a hole down the center for the two-boned beaded bracelet I was to wear until my next visit. After a few months one of these bones would join my divination set to signify me, "the *sangoma.*" I would always need to wear the other.

The circle has no sides and the spiral has no top.

Ndumbas and yurts are both round, as are many things related to indigenous wisdom. It was only when the Europeans came to Africa that squares and rectangles took over. When I returned to California, I decided to use a yurt for my *ndumba.* Yurts are very popular on the west coast and a perfect match for the circular design of the *ndumba.* Like the *ndumba,* the yurt has wooden roof supports radiating outward and downward from a central point on the dome. The roof of the yurt, however, is vinyl or canvas and not thatch. The supports have a symbolic meaning, namely that all Southern African tribes have a common core belief in spite of the plethora of different cultures in the sub-continent. The central point on the roof of the *ndumba* represents the original source from which all these arose. Belief in the ancestors is one of the most important common denominators permeating a multitude of traditions in Africa. I decided that an *ndumba* in my back yard would feel very comfortable for my African ancestors. A wooden deck was constructed and a small yurt erected on top of it. I furnished it with memorabilia of my African past with gifts for Mpofu and introduced my ancestors to their new home. I have been throwing the bones in there ever since.

The ancestors cannot save but simply alert, advise and warn,
and only according to your openness and willingness. They cannot
change or deter you from your own insistency no matter to what it's
due. Only you can choose to change. Such is the design of free will.

P.H. was correct. The bones talk! The bones read the waking dream that is the person's life. The healer is attentive to the fact that there is always free will and that anything can be changed. Bone readings are usually concerned with helping people deal with their current dilemmas—health, marital discord, money trouble, and other problems. But the bones can also warn a person not to take an upcoming journey, and they can highlight a past event that has bearing on the present. The future can always change because of free will brought to bear on the present moment. Far-reaching and accurate prophesies, therefore, are somewhat suspect, since free will is always present to shift the variables and alter the future.

If one were to ask a *sangoma* how dowsing works, she would say that the spirit was moving the dowsing stick in the direction of water. I was still to learn that *sangomas* will sometimes use special devices that "point," or indicate direction, to help them glean information from the ancestral "Field."

I was told that when I got back to California my bed was going to shake. I thought to myself, "not likely," but within days of arriving back home I was awakened by my body or my whole bed shaking. I checked the newspapers the next day and asked some friends if there had been an earthquake but there was none. The shaking occurred several more times. I no longer questioned it and assumed it was the *Umbilini*. This is the Zulu equivalent for the *Kundalini* energy that was moving up my body at night. (*Kundalini* is the primal feminine serpent-like energy, described in yoga tradition, that rests at the base of the spine and can move upward, leading to spiritual transformation.) I knew I needed to go to the river, as I had been foretold, to meet with the water spirit.

When I returned to Swaziland for the third time, I had two dreams. In the first I was at P.H.'s homestead in a room with a number of white people. I could feel powerful *Kundalini* energy moving up to my third eye. The room in which I slept was small and round, very like an *ndumba*, and was crowded with spirits with whom I lived both day and night.

In the second dream I was alone in the room and my maternal grandfather came to me and firmly shook my hand. He seemed to enter my body in the form of vibrational, *Kundalini*-like energy, after which I froze and could not cry out or see. Intuitively I heard him saying to me, "You will not get possessed!" I groped for my drum to summon the homestead, as I had been instructed to do in awake time if this were to occur. Ndoda and Nduna, P.H.'s two sons, came with everyone else following into the room. I again tried to speak but was mute and no sound came out of my mouth. I woke up, recalled the visitation, and went back to sleep.

Later that morning I lay on my mat in an altered state of awareness, somewhere between sleep and wakefulness. I had a wonderful feeling of well-being, and lights and colors suffused my visual fields. Again I felt the need to call P.H., but could not speak or move. I emerged from this trance and felt elated, as if I had indeed been possessed, but was silent. P.H. later explained, "The ancestors are telling you of what is to come." My interpretation was that because of my Jewish heritage, maybe my own ancestors would not actually possess and speak directly through me, even if they were with me in my bones and my dreams. I would be mute! P.H.'s interpretation and solution was to give me special medicine to take daily so that I could indeed speak their voice.

P.H. instructed his *sangoma* wife, Miriam, to take me to the Prophet soon after my arrival. We traveled on a dirt road north of Manzini and eventually arrived at his home, which was near a Zionist church. The Zionists, the largest Black Christian sect in Southern Africa, believe in the ancestors and also in Jesus, and in so doing bridge the gap between their indigenous spirituality and Christianity. Some are more Christian in their religious practice and others more indigenous. They too become possessed, achieving altered states of consciousness and trance that allow them to access the spirit realm or Cosmic Field, which they call God or Jesus.

Miriam and I waited in the living room until the Prophet appeared. He was going to help me meet the *unzunzu* or water spirit. The Prophet sat at a table and opened a briefcase. I could not see what was behind the lid but he took a glass of water out and asked me to put two fingers inside. He took the glass behind the case again and told me that I had powerful ancestors and a very powerful water spirit connected to me. He asked me to come back two days after Christmas with his list of special offerings for the ancestors and the water spirit, which included the special cloths I was using to dance with, which made the African ancestors more comfortable coming into my body. "*Kunda*," from the Hindu word "*Kundalini*," means something that is coiled, but it can also mean a pool. I recalled reading that a full-blown *Kundalini* experience can feel like drowning in water.

After returning to P.H.'s homestead, I dreamed I was back at the Johannesburg General Hospital, and my professor, Sonny Duplessis, the doyen of all surgeons, was there in all his awe and splendor. I was again chief resident with interns and students, one of whom was frightened and held my hand. I awoke with the same feeling of eagerness I remembered having had when I first embarked on my surgical training with him.

It was Christmas, and I was the only *thwasa* student staying with P.H. December is midsummer in the Swaziland lowveld, with temperatures above 100 degrees and the humidity making it impossible to consider steaming until after 4 p.m. Late every afternoon I steamed in P.H.'s mini-sweat lodge, which was so small there was nowhere to hide from the heat. The steaming and bathing in the *muti*-filled water afterward had a wonderful effect on me, leaving me cleansed, energized, and at peace.

Drumming every morning and evening encouraged my ancestors to reveal themselves. During the drumming I sat in the center of my room that I had made into my *ndumba*. I had arranged an altar with my bones, a few power objects and some *muti* on it. The *muti* was to burn under a cloth and then be inhaled to connect with the spirits. The altar with my divination bones was on the north side of the room. I sat in front of it facing east, with a red cloth tied around my waist (a sign of the *thwasa* state), a white cloth (the color of the ancestors) over my shoulders, and several other types of multi-patterned cloths on top of these.

As the cadence of the drumming picked up, I surprised

myself by jumping to my feet and dancing. From their excla-
mations of approval the drummers seemed just as surprised as I
was. As I moved, I felt that I was possessed. There seemed to be
a spirit within me, pressuring me, making me dance as though
I were a puppet.

Miriam, however, gave me a reality check by asking periodically, "Mr. Cumes, who are you?" I was definitely in an altered
state of consciousness, and at times in trance, but the answer
kept coming back in my own voice in English, "I am Cumes."
Even though I was dancing as if I were possessed by a spirit, my
ego self was still at least partially there, and I was determined
to let things happen in their own way and not be influenced
by outside peer forces possibly pressuring me otherwise. P.H.
had given me special black *muti* to swallow to help the ancestors speak. I did not ask what was in it, since P.H. was usually
secretive about his remedies.

I assumed P.H. was satisfied with my divining skills since he
rarely tested me now. Miriam was very attentive to my spiritual needs, and it was through her taking me back to the Prophet
that my breakthrough eventually came. Every morning I awoke,
lit mphepho, a sage-like herbal offering to call the ancestors, and
burned and inhaled the special *muti* to connect me to their presence.
I then performed my rituals, prayed, and got ready for the drumming. After drumming I would do at least an hour of yoga, breath
work (*pranayama*), various *Kundalini*-activating exercises, and then
meditate before having a light breakfast. After breakfast I drank my
"bubbles," or foam, to feed my ancestors. During the heat of the day
I would read, write, meditate, and socialize. I would also practice the
Kundalini meditations because I knew this feminine, serpent power
was the gateway to the spirit world. I had brought a lot of good
reading material to help support the left-brained side of the right-

brained experiential work I was doing. I knew that for me this was essential. I had to have a thoughtful working framework in which to place this intuitive knowledge. Every now and again I would drive into Simunye or Siteki for supplies.

I ploughed avidly through Yoga and Kabbalistic texts to see if I could find any evidence that spirit possession occurred when the *Kundalini* awakened. I could find no such references. Rather, there were differing descriptions of "entering the cosmic field" described in various ways, depending on the tradition. I did come across stories of Jewish rabbis who conversed with disincarnate teachers called *maggidim*, usually in dreams. Many famous rabbis talked to their dead teachers, but I could find no evidence of actual spirit mediumship, where the guides talked through them. Due to my Hebrew roots the idea of my ancestors talking to me, especially in dreams, felt exactly right. The fact they might possess my body did not. I began to think that my cultural bias would not allow for this experience. The oneness experience, yes, I had already had inklings of it; the Buddhist nothingness and emptiness, maybe. The Bushmen experience of Kia, or out-of-body spirit flight, I thought was attainable if I spent enough time dancing with Bushmen. But as for Grandpa coming into my body and talking, I had my doubts. I tried as best I could to put aside my skepticism and open myself up to all possibilities. My concerns were later confirmed by the high Zulu prophet or sanusi, Credo Mutwa. When I related to him grandpa's dream that I would not be possessed, he said, "Why then did P.H. not listen to your ancestors as to what was required for you? They are the ones that will determine your path." P.H. had been adamant from the beginning that possession by my own ancestors was imperative, and that only when they came through would the foreign spirits follow.

I had a strong sense that there were black African spirits hovering about, and these were the ones with whom I would work more directly. I was not averse to the idea of channeling or getting possessed by these foreign mandawe spirits, and I became quite comfortable with this thought. I also felt reassured by this subsequent teaching from the ancestors:

Mysticism resides in the mystic. The mystical is an insight into the sacred and so may be apprehended in many ways and in many manifestations. Why should we think there is just one way of shamanic healing? How could we ever know with certainty the particulars of it? Does custom not change, do words not vary even in relation to people in present time and in different places? The purpose of a healing ritual is to honor the source of the healing power and call upon its force from within and without. There are generics and even specifics that catalyze, assist and support the actualizing. Intention activates the possibilities of symbolic use and attention, and then designs and assigns its purposes. Rigidity without attention to place, time and circumstances has the rituals being served instead of them serving. Use all or any part you like of what may or may not be an ancient shamanic ritual as long as you make it your own. Add to, modify and create anew, for its mystic quality will be as a light to a candle, with you being the match. Your intention and attention provide awareness and opportunity. The choice is theirs.

Two days after Christmas, I was scheduled to go to the sacred pool with the Prophet for my encounter with the water spirit. The night before, I dreamed I was taking someone into my yurt *ndumba* in California. I turned on the light inside but it would not go on. There was a dull light present through which I could see only dimly. I asked someone to fetch a new bulb. I had prayed that night that immersion in the nzunzu's river home would be like fitting a bright light in my *ndumba*, and that my spirit would be fully awakened.

The previous October, on an Inward Bound *sangoma* trip, Marilyn, a powerful psychic, had a vision. She saw me as one of a large group of impala, no different from the rest. In the next phase of the vision, I was being draped in a zebra skin by a powerful *sangoma*, but not P.H. As he wrapped the skin around me, I turned into light. This part of her vision was my wish for the upcoming day. I remembered the divination I had received beforehand from a *sangoma* in Johannesburg: "You will need to go to the river to complete. When you have done so you will be fully qualified. A man will take you there, not P.H., and you will meet him soon."

I had packed in my car the objects the Prophet requested during my first visit to him. Miriam came back at five that morning after a night of *Femba*. She was exhausted and slept intermittently in the car as I drove. After I turned off the dirt road that led onto the highway, I saw a *hammerkop* (Afrikaans for hammerhead) on the road. It flew off and circled as I approached. The *hammerkop*, also called *impundulu* in Zulu, is a powerful, mystical bird in African lore, with a head shaped like a hammer. It is also called the Lightning Bird. It is said that if you steal its eggs or annoy it, it will make lightning strike your home. Witches sometimes make use of its magical powers. In my entire lifetime I had only rarely seen these unique creatures, usually singly and occasionally as a pair. Soon I saw two more sitting on the road, and as I approached they flew off. Since the bird is unique, I thought this must be a good omen. Three birds might have been unusual; but nine, one after the other, was extraordinary, and that is how many I counted in the space of less than 20 minutes. I was driving much too fast for it to be the same bird, but even the reappearance of the same bird on the road nine times would have been inconceivable. My expectations heightened. I thought to myself that three would have been enough of a message for most people, but my ancestors knew me too well. They had to give a sign that was strong enough to convince even my skepticism. P.H. later told me that I had nine ancestors that wanted to work with me.

We arrived at the Prophet's house and we were instructed to drive to his "brother's" home. His brother was also a Prophet — a brother in faith only, and not in blood. We waited outside the brother's *ndumba* for an hour as he dispensed *muti* to a number of people, including the local policeman. It was clear that this Zionist priest was also a competent *sangoma*, and the hut was full of plant medicines. This gave me more confidence in the ritual that was to follow. He was a large man, more muscle than fat, and reminded me of a Sumo wrestler. He wore an antelope skin draped around his generous middle as a skirt.

We drove toward the river, which we could see in the distance cascading down the cliffs into the thick bush below, where it disappeared. We met the Prophets at the end of a very bad, rutted dirt road. Beyond, the track was fit only for a four-wheel drive vehicle. We would have to walk the rest of the way. The small group went ahead and Miriam and I took up the rear. She was a large woman but walked with the grace that one sees in Africa, with the two chickens in a cardboard box perfectly balanced on her head.

The walk up alongside the river was stunningly beautiful.

We wended our way through the lush subtropical forest and arrived at a large pool nestled at the foot of a waterfall. There had been a lot of rain, and the waterfall and river were in spate. At the pool I was instructed to strip down to my shorts. I set the five different colored candles on a rock and lit them. A fire had already been made. The "brother," who seemed to be the senior, rubbed my dancing cloths in the ashes. He sprayed alcohol over me and threw the rest of the contents into the pool. I took the 10 silver coins I had been told to bring to the pool edge and prayed to my ancestors, asking them to give me the light that I needed to become a more complete healer. With each invocation I threw a coin into the pool.

The chickens were being sacrificed as I was led to the water. The trunk and skeleton of a dead tree stuck out of the water's edge between some rocks. The Prophet tied a sturdy blue rope in a loop around the trunk and told me to get into the pool and hold the rope. I was ordered not to let go under any circumstances or I might be taken by the water spirit. It occurred to me that maybe at one time a *thwasa* student had a *Kundalini* experience in the pool and because of the overwhelming impulse of energy traversing the body had submerged, never to be seen again. However, now, especially after the nine lightning birds, I was more inclined to believe that just as there were terrestrial and cosmic spirits, there were water spirits, too. I obeyed the rules and held fast to the rope. The Prophet, dressed in a red tunic, got into the pool with me while the other held the rope and perched himself agilely in the dead tree.

By now the two of them were clearly in trance as they called out to Moses, the Prophets, Jesus, Jehovah, and many other names in Siswati that I did not recognize. I was overwhelmed with the power of the invocation. As they prayed, they slapped the water vigorously. Their pleas to the spirits were punctuated by thrusting my head periodically into the pool, immersing me completely. When I came up they would smack me about the arms, chest, back, shoulders, neck, head and face with some force. They were pulling back their slaps; otherwise I would have been knocked senseless, since they were both powerful men. I lost all sense of time.

Eventually I was instructed to get out of the water. I emerged dazed and staggered onto a rock, moving at first on all fours so that I did not fall over. I was trembling and felt *Kundalini* energy like electricity coursing up my body. It was a more powerful manifestation of the unmistakable feeling that had been stalking me these last few months in my dreams and in my meditations.

Miriam took my place in the pool, and I noted a look of terror on her face as she entered, perhaps in fear of the *unzunzu*. She underwent the same ritual as I had, in her case to revisit the water spirit. When she came out of the pool, I saw an approving look from her and the Prophet as I shuddered, trembled and shook while the serpent power granted by the *unzunzu* moved up my body. Along with the energy was a sense of euphoria and oneness. I felt tears welling up, together with the sensation of absolute peace and contentment. Everything around me looked different. There was a numinous glow wherever I turned my gaze.

I washed from top to toe with the bucket full of water, chicken blood, and *muti*, and poured the rest over my head. Then I rinsed off in the river and stumbled back onto the rock to dry off in the sun, bewildered but ecstatic. The ceremony was complete except for the offering of the cooked chicken, pieces of which I had to spit in all four directions. Finally I savored some of the meat before walking down the hill to the car. I had been instructed not to look back, and I felt as if I might be in a dream from the Old Testament. Miriam told me to drive back to the brother's home. She had to get special *muti* from the water spirit for me and for her. This was the new *muti* that I would use for my steaming.

After the day at the pool, I felt I had undergone a transformation, as if some new force had taken hold inside me. In the evening during the drumming, I felt myself shake and convulse as I had at the pool. I would spring up and dance, but when I sat down and P.H. asked me to identify myself, there was a different response. "I am Job," I heard myself saying. I was still aware of being David Cumes, but it was as if the voice that was mine was coming from another source and was directed toward me as it spoke. I was still there, I was speaking in my own voice, but I felt that I had moved aside, that it was not I who was conversing. I realized that I was channeling Job, an old Zulu who worked for my family when I was a small boy and who had been like a father to me. It was Job who had taught me to ride a bike, how to make a spear, and how to throw it. Job had magnified my boyhood images of Africa.

P.H. asked again, "Who are you?"

Job responded, "I am an old Zulu who was a friend of Cumes. I helped in his house."

"How are you here to help?" P.H. inquired. "Are you a healer?"

"I am not a healer. He is already a healer and can heal. I am a pure Zulu spirit and can help him be straight on his path. I can give him energy so that his hands can heal through God. I like to dance, and his body will be free if I dance him, and this will make him a better healer."

A few days before Job spoke, I had sensed that there was a spirit close to me. I knew I had not fabricated Job, since I had not thought of him in years. I had, however, thought about Samuel in the recent past. Samuel had been a *sangoma* who had worked in our household some time after Job had returned home to his wives, children, homestead and cattle. I had also been very fond of Samuel. If my subconscious had contrived someone to channel in advance it would have been Samuel, the *sangoma*, and not Job. Because I am somewhat cynical, I often look for reasons that my subconscious would sabotage a "real" experience. I could not find one here. Job's name came to me from a far-off place during the beats of the drum. P.H. had said that I must not think, that I should just say what arose spontaneously in my mind, and that would then be the ancestor. These spirits would be identified by a name that popped into my head. P.H. now thought that maybe Job would be the leader and would show the way for the other ancestors. My ancestors, not being familiar with the tradition, might defer to him. P.H. explained that other foreign spirits that I did not know might also come.

That night I dreamt a Celtic tune, which I sang in my dream state. The name Daniel came to me in my reverie, and I wondered if Daniel were another guide. I was awakened by the sound of drums in the hallway outside my closed door. I sat up to be sure I was really awake and not dreaming. The sound of the drums was unmistakable and there was shuffling in the hallway and then in the adjacent bathroom. I called out, "Who is it?" There was no reply. I got up and opened the door. The hallway was empty except for the drums, but there were no drummers beating on them. I checked the two outside doors to the building; both were locked from the inside. I decided it must be Daniel and that he must like to drum. When I asked P.H. about this the next morning he said, "Of course it's Daniel. He is another foreign guide. Who else do you think this could be?" He confirmed that Daniel might be Irish or Scottish and liked to drum.

At five a.m. Miriam arrived for the morning session. With the drumming I smelled a distinct odor, which I remembered smelling in my dream the night before. I shook and convulsed. A spirit seemed to be coming through. I got up to dance but the internal force impelling me to move did not feel that he belonged to the dance so I sat down and moved to the sound of the drums, which felt appropriate. The familiar convulsive wave passing up my body, up my back and spine to the shoulders, neck and head reassured me that I was in touch with the *Kundalini*. The energy was different this time, and the smell made me say "Daniel" when P.H. asked him to identify himself.

"Why are you here?" P.H. asked.

"I have come to free him from his cage so that he can be a better healer. The reason he likes Celtic music and feels it inside is because of me."

"Are you a healer?" again from P.H.

"No, but I can help him be a better one by freeing him."

It seemed I was locked in, a victim of my past conditioning, and now two guides were there to help me get out. Daniel liked to drum and enjoyed moving to the voice of the drum. He was less interested in dancing. P.H. was pleased that two guides had come through. On another night, I heard drumming coming from the drum next to me while I tried to fall asleep. This time I knew it was Daniel and politely asked him to go away and let me sleep. Later on, more Celtic spirit guides were to appear, but I did not experience Daniel again after I returned to California.

Now the foundations of indigenous healing, and especially ancestral possession and channeling, which had previously sounded so strange to me, took on new meaning. My actual experience of them reinforced my decision to complete my initiation and fully pursue this new calling. I felt that I had finally "arrived"! The next day, although I was awake, I felt I was in a dream state. I had heard the term "a house of dreams" applied to aspects of the *thwasa* experience. When I lay down I felt butterflies in my heart, and when I closed my eyes I saw vivid light patterns.

The day I was due to return to Johannesburg, there was powerful drumming in the morning session to make more ancestors reveal themselves. Up until then I had been surprised that my main ancestor, Mpofu, had not yet appeared. Although I felt her presence whenever I threw bones, I had never had direct communication with her, except once in a dream. A *sangoma* earlier had told me that if a beautiful woman who was soft, kind, and gentle appeared in my dreams, it would be Mpofu, and it was in this way that she had presented herself previously in a dream, carrying three traditional drums.

That day I sensed another presence and asked the question, "Mpofu, are you there?"

The answer came back, "Who do you think has been here with you and the bones all this time?"

P.H. asked Mpofu, "What can we do to help this man?"

"You can strengthen his bones," she replied. "There is no one to drum for him in California, and if he became fully possessed they would think him mad. Only the bones will make him believable there." P.H. dutifully gave me special *muti* for the bones along with other remedies before I left, and I think silently acknowledged that frank spirit possession would not be my path. My work would be through the bones, dreams and plant medicines. I agreed with Mpofu and doubted that my status as a surgeon would allow for possession, or its more user-friendly term, trance-channeling, even in California.

It was around this time that I connected with a different part of South Africa. I was drawn to Limpopo, where I had encountered many powerful *sangomas* on Inward Bound trips I had facilitated. One of these, Andries, had especially impressed me, and I decided it was time to take my healing path to the next level. P.H. had remained adamant that I continue to work towards my own ancestors coming through, but I had learned otherwise from Credo Mutwa, who was the last word when it came to African healing wisdom. Moses Shado Dudlu, another powerful *sangoma* and mentor to me from the beginning of my journey, had also divined and affirmed I was now complete, except for one thing. I knew nothing about *muti*, and I needed to learn this.

It was Andries who eventually tested me and finalized my initiation by graduating me. He gave me the necessary necklaces and amulets and an armamentarium of medicinal plants to work with until such time as I knew how to collect my own. My diagnostic skills were finely tuned, he said, but I had no "medicine bag." He provided me with one in the meantime. He was clear that we would be working together from now on, and he was certain Limpopo would be my new home away from home. He told me I was free to practice and that I should be supremely confident in my abilities because my spirit had been fully activated, and the ancestors were with me. Not only was I awarded the *sangoma* ware to go along with my new status and a pharmacopoeia to complement my diagnostic bones,

I was also given what I feel is the ultimate compliment by this elderly Tsonga master. "You are *ndoda nyama*," he said, "You are a black man." I never realized how true this was until a later time when my ancestors revealed to me that I had been a black man in two previous incarnations.

My next task was to learn spirit medicines, or *muti*. I felt as if I had just completed medical school and now had to complete not only an "internship" but also some postgraduate training in the form of a "*sangoma* residency." My journey had just begun.

One does not treat an ailment but rather the person.
The same symptoms may be treated radically differently
in different people. Herbal remedies are not selected and
employed solely for the healing power of the herb itself but
also for its ability to awaken the dormant healing power
that everybody has, or to reinforce the already aroused
healing capacity of the patient.
Rituals and practices will vary even as people do.
What today is called the placebo effect does not imply
fooling the patient into believing in something that is not,
but rather in medicating him with faith in what could
happen if allowed.
A person's skepticism, anxiety and dismay may impair
the healing and stand in the way of his
activating his own inner healer.
As soon as the patient becomes open to the possibility of the
treatment's efficacy, be it a ritual, an herb or a suggestion;
hope and then belief work their own magic.

III

The Kabbalistic & Celtic connection

Your God-given destiny is the hunt of your life.
Hold to the scent, stay on the spoor.

You can only be you. What does not encourage, nourish
and advance can only divert, feed upon and distract. You
have to find the way designated to you by God.

Do not tarry, pay attention carefully
to how you choose to fill your hour.

The value of information is in its being
used for transformation.

Humility is truthful acknowledgment about the wonders
of yourself, taking appropriate credit for your part,
while recognizing God's gifts to you.

IN 1998, BEFORE MY INITIATION, I FIRST MET MARYELLEN KELLEY. She headed up the Omega program of Santa Barbara's adult education program and also had significant status as a senior citizen in the community. I began facilitating workshops for her programs, which spoke to the subjects of my first two books and had to do with the general principles of healing, especially pertaining to the power of nature or wilderness as healer. Once I began my *Thwasa*, I also began to lecture on ancient indigenous healing methods, and later, on dreams. We became friends and would meet frequently to talk about upcoming teaching sessions. I had become frustrated by the limitations of allopathic medicine and was on a quest to find an alternative healing paradigm. Her Omega programs became an ideal forum for me to voice some of the ideas that I wanted to express. Thus began a fifteen-year friendship and working relationship.

Around this time Maryellen began to have dreams for me from various ancestral personages she did not know. Ancestors, being very practical, will use the most accessible channel, and Maryellen appeared to be uniquely gifted in this regard. The array of personalities coming into her dreamscape was staggering – Hebrew, African, Celtic, animal, mythical and otherwise. This talent was previously unbeknown to her. Although I would have most of my dreams in metaphor and an occasional ancestral visitation, she began to experience visits from a host of different spirit guides who seemed to want to send us information. Later on it became clear that she and I were destined in some way to work together on behalf of a litany of ancestors that represented the universal truths of three wisdoms – African, Kabbalistic and Celtic. At the same time I began to receive original songs in my dreams from similar genres of music. This is addressed in a later chapter.

One day when we met to discuss future topics for Omega's programs, she told me that an elderly man had appeared in her dreams whom, after her description, I thought might be my grandfather. Shortly after that, a tall, jolly, dark and robust man with a pleasant body scent showed up with my "grandfather," and was accompanied by a dog who, in the dream, was called "White

Dog" for obvious reasons. Her description of this man sounded very much like my favorite uncle, Sam, including my fond remembrance of his unique and pleasant body odor. The next time we met, I brought along the family photo album, and saying nothing, allowed her to page through it. Without any hesitation she identified the grandfather on my mother's side and my uncle Sam, his son. I was astonished. Hence I became reacquainted with them both during my *Thwasa* and through Maryellen.

I had never known my grandfather; he had died long before I was born. My mother had spoken of him frequently, saying how much I reminded her of him. I now know that we can be loved by ancestors on the other side even if we have never known them in this lifetime. These ancestors, indeed, may well have been our mothers, fathers, sisters, brothers, friends or lovers in past lives. Hence the love bond and their desire to be of help to us as spirit guides. The Buddhists have a practice in which they regard everyone they meet with the same love and compassion as they would if that person had been their mother. This makes a lot of spiritual sense. It is feasible, due to the fact we all cycle in and out of various lifetimes, that such a person could well have been one's mother or similar close relative or loved one. Love is the catalyst that allows them to more easily cross the veil between worlds to visit us in dreams. One of the first things that Grandpa told Maryellen was,

"Tell him there is the vision for the appointed time. If it seems to tarry he must wait for it patiently. It will surely come. It will not delay. It will reveal as it should."

At a later date a dark, tall, imposing patriarch began to appear. Dressed in a white robe, he looked like someone out of a remote biblical epoch. I recalled a sacred ceremony in the Amazon jungle years previously in which the curandero or shaman who was in trance said he could see a biblical-like figure dressed in a white robe close to me. The image was associated with the symbols of a menorah and a caduceus. He deduced from this that there was a Jewish physician amongst the small group involved in the healing ceremony. This man's name, Maryellen told me, was Isea.

After this a number of other Kabbalistic characters began to show themselves, whom she was told were *Tzaddikim*, which could loosely be translated as enlightened or righteous ones. Over the next several years it became apparent that P.H. had miscalculated, and there were many more than nine spirit guides who seemed interested in the work that Maryellen and I were to do together in the future. It seemed to me that now that I was a *sangoma* I had become visible to certain guides on the other side of the veil, or *pargawd*, as it is called in Kabbalah. I was mystified. I assumed that because of my newly acquired *sangoma* status, my past lives and my roots, we had been admitted through the back door, or servant's entrance if you like, into a higher mystical realm.

It took Maryellen and me several years of tutoring from the other side to take all this seriously. Her description of the two of us showing up in the guise of Minnie and Mickey Mouse among these *Tzaddikim* appeared to make the most sense to us at that time. Anselm, Isaac, Arn, a stunning black woman called Tumutu, and a black man of Lemba origin called James now joined Mpofu, Grandpa, Sam and Isea. There were more to follow, but of note were three Celtic guides: Malachy, Mac and Caleb by name. All were joined by another Kabbalist called Mo. Mo taught in a formal way. He would show up in dreams in which Maryellen and I sat at desks in a classroom, and he would instruct us on various aspects of secret wisdom. Although I was present in the dreams, I would have no conscious recollection of them the next day. I was reassured that the knowledge nevertheless resided in my subconscious. Maryellen, on the other hand, would wake up from the dream and write down each minute detail, which we would read together again and again over the years. There were other less formal teachings that came sporadically from other guides as well. In 2012 these culminated in a small book of sayings entitled *Messages from the Ancestors – Wisdom for the Way.* Some of these are interspersed throughout this text, along with others. They can also be regarded in some ways like koans for meditation, with many levels of understanding. These and other teachings have impacted our lives and brought new levels of meaning to the *sangoma* wisdom I had already been taught. We trust those included in the text will also edify and inform you as they have us.

IV

Ancestors and the Dream world

*Visitations, like the bones, manifest outside the dream
state. They too alert, inform, advise, guide, comfort or
directly engage, but unlike the bones, they cannot be
called upon at will. They are rare in occurrence but can
be abundant and concentrated when the visitors
feel a sense of urgency, wantfulness, insistence and have
the ability and will to transcend the difficulties.
Visitations take enormous energy and have other limiting
factors as well and so are prompted by great purpose
and seek open, accessible conduits.
Be careful of saying, "just a dream" or "only a dream."
In attempting to distinguish between what is real and
what is not, we would do just as well to say, "it was just
awake time … It was only awake time."
The dream time is not less real, it is simply a different
mode of being, of learning, of expressing, and one where
the guardedness and contrived-ness of ego is relaxed.
We must remember we only come here to dream.
We only come here to sleep.*

"It is not true, it is not true that we come to earth to live!"
Pre-Columbian saying

THE WAY MY LIFE UNFOLDED AFTER THE INITIATION CANNOT be separated from the dream world that pervaded my consciousness on certain nights. I would not have found Tshismane healing center if not for a "Big" dream followed by a series of follow-up dreams. Furthermore, I would not have eventually left it after its completion if not for a series of profound warning dreams. Added to this was the dream guidance coming from others as well. Hence a few words need to be said about an indigenous approach to the dream world.

For some of us, the easiest form of access to the cosmic infinity and to realms not localized in space and time is the dream world. According to the *sangomas*, our dream state is every bit as real as the waking state. All we have to do is decipher the cosmic conversation. We have to understand the metaphors and the passwords. These symbols may be highly individual, and it is up to each one of us to find our own individual code. The ancestral "Field" has a particular dialogue for each person that depends on their blood root, their culture, their religion and their education. When we learn to encourage our dreams and understand the conversation, we open up to a user-friendly source of wonder and sometimes life-saving information.

Dreams can be very puzzling and convoluted, and their purpose does not always reveal itself immediately. One may have to search deeply and long for more meaning. Frequently I have received a message that seemed trivial or insignificant only to find later that it proved profoundly accurate. The same can be true for the divining bones that read the waking dream that is the individual's life. It is important to know that neither the dreams nor the bones are localized in space and time, and that a prophetic dream or truth from a bone divination may precede the event by many years. There is no time on the other side of the veil and this sometimes accounts for the temporal delay.

Long ago and the future will meet to know
themselves as one.

The ancestors work in strange ways. Sometimes the dreams are literal, sometimes not. One *sangoma* told me that there are basically two types of dreams: instructional and non-instructional. Sometimes we are being told something directly, and if we ignore the instructions we may never find the message that is waiting for us or identify the danger that lurks. The ancestors, or whatever we wish to call the information "Field," usually work in metaphor, and often we need to unravel the secret. Important dreams often have a different quality, a heightened intensity; they alert us to the fact that we may be receiving an official communication from the spirit world.

There are numerous fine books written by gifted dream interpreters. Most of these speak to the dream coming to the dreamer out of the subconscious. However, dreams are also a personal phenomenon, individual expressions, often of universal truths, or messages that come in the night to tell us of something we need to know. These can be scripted by a source outside of our consciousness or subconscious by our spirit guides. If one is astute and keeps a record, one can see patterns emerge that can assist us in the interpretation of our dreams without using scholarly research to unravel them. In my case I seem to be able to characterize these consistent dream themes as visitations, empowerments, warnings, nudgings, instructions, affirmations, acts of a play (usually prophetic), luminous and numinous (usually "Big" dreams), those associated with bodily vibrations, dream songs or words as messages, "getting someone else's mail," and dreams that speak in tongues. We each have our own unique way of dreaming, so what applies to me may not apply to others. It is up to each of us to discover our own particular dream code. These indigenous principles, therefore, are just to guide and give a different approach to looking at them.

A visitation is not really a dream but rather a true visit from a spirit guide, or sometimes an intrusive entity. The former are infrequent and require a tremendous effort on the part of the spirit. The more the information conveyed, and the more the detail, the more the energy required on the part of the ancestor. This is why they are occasions for much gratitude. Maryellen is a particularly gifted channel that appears to receive these visits in exquisite detail.

Of course not all the dreams are messages or instructions from the ancestors. Some may make no sense, others are helpful, and some are life-saving. The question – and the challenge – are how to recognize those instructional dreams and interpret them. The "garbage" dreams of the night may be the subconscious playing itself out. They are often related to some event that has occurred in the recent past that triggers the image. Nightmares sometimes fit into this category, and they may be generated by fear or by one's sense of physical discomfort while asleep. For instance if I am too hot, I am more apt to have nightmares. If I need to empty my bladder, I have dreams of being in search of a bathroom. Watching a scary movie in the evening may engender terrifying dreams. This may be because of being pulled into a dark dream "vibration" or reality initiated during an inharmonious and unsettling awake state. This is why I prefer to avoid images and news that could either affect my psyche or drag my consciousness or dream body down into an undesirable realm. We really do create our own consciousness, both when we are awake and when we are asleep.

On the other hand, the ancestors may be inclined to use recent images to convey a warning. For instance, a dream of being drowned by a tsunami may be an admonition that something is about to occur that could "drown" you health-wise or financially.

The nightmare is frequently a "Big" dream sent to get one's immediate attention. The energy in the dream may be overstated so that we will be alerted to something that can be avoided if the correct steps are taken.

Apparition dreams, such as a face or the figure of a person, sometimes in white, occur at times. These dreams are often prophetic and may warn of something bad to come. For instance, on a trip into the Amazon jungle I had a phantom dream of a friend whom I had not seen for years. He was an orthopedic surgeon who had a unique way of fixing a certain type of wrist fracture. Early the next morning I fell off a high platform in the jungle and sustained the very same fracture I so closely associated with him. Sadly, I only remembered the warning dream after the fact, while nursing my broken arm on the trip out of the jungle for medical attention.

The most prophetic kind of dream is the rarest. For me it usually presents as a profound, vivid series of events, often like three or more scenes of a play. The information that "plays out" is so striking that it cannot be ignored. These dreams often portend the future in some detail. A few years before my marriage split up, I had a vivid dream as to how this rupture would unfold, all of which came true. After we divorced, I had another dream of the magnificent garden of the home we had shared.

All the trees and shrubs had been cut down, and the garden was devastated. However, when I looked at the rich brown earth beneath the rubble, water was bubbling out and new seeds were sprouting everywhere. The dream told me that the future for both of us would be fertile and fruitful, which proved to be true. These dreams are palpably different in character and have a numinous or luminous, sometimes Technicolor quality to them. One knows immediately upon awakening that they are important.

Today, many people cannot believe that God, or anyone else from beyond our own realm, speaks to us. We think that prophetic, biblical-style dreams no longer occur as actual instruments of prophecy. This is not true. We may not have the same kind of prophetic dreams as Pharaoh that reveal the future of an entire people. However, we do receive important personal messages that can help ease our way through life and keep us in line with our destiny path. At the very least, we awaken with the sense that we are being supported from another domain. The *sangomas* appreciate that ancestral dreams usually occur in the early morning. They say this is when the ancestors are active. The fact that physiologists would say this is the period of REM or rapid eye movement sleep does not exclude the possibility that guiding forces may be present.

Usually our dream world is a little thing in the grand scheme of world events, though it is often critical for ourselves and our life's journey. There can be many variables, and free will is forever present to shift each variable. Prophesy, therefore, can be especially tricky if it encompasses the future of a whole nation or relates to world affairs. Also one has to be sure that it is not a trickster that is scripting the dream to sabotage one's progress.

Aboriginal peoples hold great store in dreams because they

know how to use them. The knowledge gained is verifiable as time comes to pass. *Sangomas* dream about patients coming to them and about specific plant remedies for those patients. Even though they may never have seen that particular plant before, they will go into the bush, find it, and then dispense it.

Sometimes my dreams are associated with a sensation of vibrational energy that permeates my body. This association with *Kundalini* energy is, for me, an endorsement of the validity of the message.

Sometimes I dream a song, a sentence or even written text. Occasionally it is a song that I know, and the message is in the words of the song. At other times I dream a tune that is haunting, original, and quite beautiful, sometimes even celestial. In my half-awake state after the dream, I go over it and record it on a recorder (now my smart phone) I have next to my bed. On other occasions I have dreamed written text. I also dreamt the wording of the titles of two of my books. Occasionally I will hear a voice that gives me short and concise information that is sometimes a warning or highly meaningful. *For example, "God is not a test of love – God's love is not a test!"*

I recently gave a talk on Soul Loss, which occurs when a person is disconnected from his or her own predestined higher purpose. The night before, while dreaming, I heard a voice say two words, "Destiny! Accountability!" After the dream I changed the content of the lecture to include these key concepts that I had omitted. On a more recent occasion I had this sentence before a talk where the topic of judgment was key: *"At the end of the day, when you no longer need to be right, the essence of your soul will shine through."*

There are dreams that close friends, relations or loved ones may have on our behalf. These can also be prophetic and can sometimes predict illness or even death. I had an apparition of a favorite aunt's face shortly before she died. Maryellen and my business manager, Adrienne, frequently relate warning dreams to me to keep me out of trouble. Adrienne once dreamed about a piece of property I was fixated on buying for a wilderness retreat in Santa Barbara County a few years before my *sangoma* initiation. In her dream, the entire cliff on which the proposed parcel was located fell away in a huge landslide, carrying me with it. When she found me at the bottom of the hill I was dead and my body was bloated. Several weeks after her dream, there was a significant slide on that piece of land. In this case the dream came true, but the land "slide" was also a warning against a bad real estate decision and a critical "fall."

It seems that when the ancestors feel they are being ignored, they will resort to sending a stronger message to you via someone else who has influence. Sometimes these come with foreign words that only the one for whom the dream is intended can understand. This is because the spirits want to lend emphasis to the message. This form of dream telling is called "getting someone else's mail."

Concerning those who dream for others. They help to get your attention in a way that could not be commanded otherwise. The senders use what they feel is the most effective way of advising, enlightening, warning and encouraging. Sometimes, just to make you feel supported and loved, devices are used that you cannot easily dismiss.

When I first met Maryellen, although I was very much steeped in the *sangoma* dream paradigm, I always kept a healthy skepticism about "spiritual messages" both for myself and certainly from others. The ancestors, knowing this, would send messages in Zulu, Afrikaans and Hebrew, none of which she understood but would write out phonetically. This reassured me that the dreams were coming from an ancestral source outside of Maryellen's psyche and I took them to heart.

Aboriginal people, and others who are closer to nature, will often dream about the health of the environment or have dreams that come from their animal spirit helpers or power animals. These same animals can present themselves in awake time to guide or warn of what is ahead on the journey or just to support.

I find it helpful to classify my dreams in the following main categories before logging them into my computer dream journal: VISITATIONS, WARNINGS, EMPOWERMENTS, NUDGINGS, INSTRUCTIONS, SONGS AND SAYINGS, POWER ANIMALS and those that we are not sure of, DREAMS TO TEND (an important category credited to the dream expert Steven Eisenstadt).

We are all given dreams for a purpose, and one should not need years of special training in order to interpret them. Maryellen, when she first asked me to start lecturing on dreams, said to me, "Dreams are far too important to be relegated to experts." I supposed this might be considered a backhanded compliment, but it gave me the impetus to begin lecturing on an indigenous approach to dreams, in spite of not being able to lay claim to any formal psychological training on the subject. The ancestors affirmed Maryellen's wisdom:

*A psychological orientation that explains dreams as
scripted only by the subconscious makes dream
interpretation quite limited.*

It is clear, however, that one has to translate the dream metaphor into something that fits the dreamer's own particular psyche, culture, religion, education and conditioning, and not necessarily that of a psychologist or anyone else. For instance if a Christian were to dream of fish this might have religious symbolism. If a Venda person were to have a fish dream he might interpret it as having to do with receiving money rather than grace. To a Zulu, dreaming of a dog might mean witchcraft, whereas to a dog lover it may speak of loyalty and unconditional love. If we have difficulty with the interpretation, an intuitive outsider can be invaluable in keeping us close to the truth. Ego, self-denial or lack of insight, however, can trip us all up.

When we seek the help of others in interpretation it is important that we look to their spirituality as it is to our own for clarity. Those with a high level of spirituality are able to activate positive energy even from the most negative dream.

If nothing else, we can remember that instructional dreams can come from the spirit world to help, warn, nudge and guide us. Sometimes we ignore the instructions at our own peril. It is not always so much that one acts on a single dream, but rather on a pattern of many dreams. It is also true that some dreams are so compelling that they force us to pay attention to their specifics. Dreams, rather than being the absolute truth of that moment, may be signposts to guide us along our way. Furthermore, when one sees or experiences something in waking life that has already been encountered in a dream, it cannot be ignored as easily.

Some dreams are powerful because, while they relate to us, they are not prompted by specific recent events such as conversations, meetings, movies, and so on, nor are they reflections of our hopes and fears about such incidents or conditions. Instead it is their detachment from ego and our daily lives that gives these dreams the capacity to lead us to the truth. However, the opposite is also true:

> *A person is shown what is suggested by the*
> *reflections of his mind and this is why we take*
> *from dreams positive messages, enlightening*
> *thoughts and happy feelings,*
> *because they find a welcome in our mind-set*
> *and emotions. Others, however, disturb*
> *our equanimity with doubts and fears.*

One Kabbalist who spent years studying with his master was asked what he learned in all that time. He replied, "I learned how to sleep." The dream world and the *sangoma's* world are inseparable, and after my initiation the ancestors began teaching me how to sleep.

Around that time I had a voice in a dream that said to me, "the snake brings the dream." This emphasized the importance of spiritual practice to the dream time. The *Kundalini*, serpent, feminine energy needs coaxing from its hiding place in order to open up the third eye or sixth chakra for dreaming. Hence during the drumming and dancing of my *Thwasa*, my dreams were most prolific. The same thing can occur with extended retreats into wild places.

The bones reveal the waking dream that is a person's life, and interpretations offered by the *sangomas* are offered very humbly and democratically. For instance, in the bones "money" can also represent energy. Hence if the bones reveal that a patient is "broke" money-wise, this could also mean he or she is energy depleted or "burnt out." It is up to the client to tell the *sangoma* which of these it is. Similarly, dream interpretation should always be offered with caution and humility. The dreamer is the final arbitrator of his dream.

The most skillful interpreter, even one who knows you
well, can at best only be revealing, suggesting and guiding.

I have been warned by the ancestors not to make my interpretation of the dream fit what I would like it to mean, rather than attending to the nudging or the warning the ancestors are trying to convey to put me on the correct path. This is why it may sometimes be difficult to dissect out the meaning of one's own dream and be objective about it, especially when the stakes are high for a particular desired outcome. The same is true for bone divination, and this why many *sangomas* will not do divinations for themselves.

Beware of making the interpretation of the
dream fit to what the ego desires.

If we have our own agenda aside from what the dream is telling us, we may not take the appropriate action. If we do not, the consequences can be serious. However, if we are able to discern the message accurately we will be able to abort an unpleasant or even dangerous outcome. Similarly, the bones tell us "what to see," but because of free will they cannot say "what we must be." Only we can decide that.

Dreams speak not to the way things have to be, but to the way they will be unless action is taken. The dream outcome can always be altered, as can the prognosis of a bone divination.

Free will, which we can all act upon, is the cosmic law.

We also have to appreciate that trickster spirits and dark forces have access to our dream world. This is somewhat analogous to the Internet. The magic of Google can help us on our life path, but there are also viruses, Trojan horses, pornographic pop-ups and all sorts of negative and even demonic-like "intruders" that can corrupt our dream files and change the context of the message. Their purpose is to confuse us and take us away from the path of truth. This is why sometimes the ancestors have to resort to devious dream metaphors in order to bypass the spyware of the dark forces. Hence the ancestors advised that ...

The dark forces can intrude in dreams but keep in mind
that distortions may also be projections of your own fears,
doubts, insecurities and questions about yourself as well.
Furthermore, the dark forces relish using
such to your disadvantage, confusion and alienation.
You cannot have a dream without false imaginings and
interminglings. Parts are true and parts are false. There
is no dream that does not reflect both this side and that.
Demonic forces and tricksters lurk to smuggle false images
and messages into the dreams.
Many truths are revealed in dreams, but be alert to falsities
as well, most especially in interpretation.

Dream interpretation can be difficult and also carries with it a heavy responsibility, since the interpretation of the dream, right or wrong, has the power to actualize the outcome. The same is true of bone divination, which can create an adverse outcome if the display is poorly interpreted.

The dream follows its interpretation.

*Dreams contain both truth and lies, and hence the words
of the interpretation prevail over everything in that they
determine whether the true or false part will prevail.
All symbols in a dream have potential energy, and it is
the interpretation that activates it.
The interpretation assigns its manifestation, and that
potential can be actualized either way.
How can we be sure that we are not interpreting wrongly
and thus impacting ourselves or the world negatively?
Ego is the biggest stumbling block encompassing expectations
of ourselves and others.
Also competing for attention are our fears, worries, guilts
and resentments. The more we are aware of these traits,
tendencies and weaknesses the easier it is to avoid interpretations
that cater to them.
A spiritual focus is our truest guide.*

*Just as the use of a tool is its value, so is interpretation
what gives importance to a dream. The way a dream is
interpreted is the way it will come to pass in the material
world. The very interpretation can become a self-fulfilling
prophecy and has potential to play itself out.*

V

spirit songs from the Dream world

WHEN I BEGAN MY INITIATION AT THE TURN OF THE millennium, I began to get songs in my dreams. These presented in different ways, such as choirs singing, musicians playing, people dancing, a dream sequence manifesting on a TV screen, and in other odd ways. Most commonly I would just wake up with a song in my head. Some of the songs were celestial, others very special, some really good and many quite ordinary. On awakening, I would record them on a device that I kept next to my bed. More recently I have begun to get tunes in awake time, long after I have gotten out of bed.

I would share them with Maryellen, who had two friends with a recording studio, and in the beginning we would record them in a raw state at their studio. I shared these with intimate friends who were struck by the strange way I was receiving them, but who were not very impressed with the raw recordings. I, however, was convinced of their value, but not of my ability to do them justice. I would tell Maryellen that I needed to find the right musician to do the job well, but she was convinced that I was to be the singer. Although I can hold a tune, I have no musical knowledge whatsoever, and not much talent.

After months of frustration, a musician friend in South Africa told me about Eugene Havenga, whom he intuitively felt was the right person to help me. Eugene has a distinct spiritual inclination, but I was still surprised, after giving him a sample of the songs to review, when he said the following: "Dave, these are very special, but you must be the one to sing them. I can help with the arranging and harmonizing, but the songs were meant for you and you must be the artist." When I told Maryellen this she gloated shamelessly and said, "I told you so!"

I was still unconvinced, but decided to proceed with Eugene, who at the time was living in a remote spiritual community in the north of South Africa close to a little town called Duiwelskloof (Devil's Cliff). Eugene is a gifted musician who had fallen on hard times and bad health and was rehabilitating in this remote spot. He is a superb guitarist and drummer, and he also had a sophisticated computer system with a keyboard that allowed us to choose the right instruments for any particular song. There were many different genres of songs that I was getting: African, Celtic, Chassidic, Native American and others. I assumed at the time that, for some obscure reason, I had the ability to retain these often complex rhythms in my dream psyche, and that was the reason I was channeling them from a host of different spirit cultures. I guessed that maybe they were coming from frustrated, deceased, talented musicians who now were taking the opportunity to once again have their songs produced even though they had been long gone from the planet. I had always believed that a strong affinity for a certain music genre was a guide to which past lives we might have had. I was very partial to music from all of these cultures. It occurred to me that the amazing celestial-like songs I sometimes heard may have been coming from "the music of the spheres." Mac, one of the Celtic ancestors, once appeared to Maryellen in a dream and suggested that there were times I was tuning into the sacred tune of the universe or *Oran Mor* – Celtic for the music that fills all creation with its divine harmony, which sounds similar to the description of the "music of the spheres."

I assumed the songs were for healing, dreaming and meditating, since they were so unique. Many were chants, some had words that were messages, and others had some phrases but needed lyrics to be added for completion. Early on in this experience, when I would get a chant, Maryellen would dream Zulu or Hebrew words that I would put to the chant, assuming they were meant to go together. There were times also that she would dream the rest of the lyrics to the first line or two I had received that week. At the time of this writing I have more than a 250 songs that have been mastered onto nineteen CDs, and more still keep on coming. There are still hundreds that have not been attended, though most of the best ones have been done.

Whenever I go back to South Africa, I include several weeks with Eugene and we usually manage up to twenty songs at a time. I continue to return, at least yearly, to South Africa to work with Eugene. He has now moved to Johannesburg where his talent can be better appreciated. We have taken the music to another level as we have learned to work better together and, especially, with the ancestors, and also because the songs are increasing in complexity. Eugene is very tuned in to the spirit world when we are together, and he gets messages from them both in the dream and awake time as to how to arrange the music.

As the compositions began to improve, so too did the interference from trickster spirits increase. Music can reflect both dark and light, and there is more than enough dark music on the planet today with the likes of some heavy metal and rap. It sometimes seemed that the dark forces were keen to sabotage our renderings, mainly because the vibration of the music was very refined and they did not like this.

The interference would manifest in many ways. It was not uncommon that when I would arrive, or during my stay, for some unexplained reason the computer would just crash. Eugene would get his technical expert to come out and usually nothing wrong could be found. On other occasions, songs that had been saved to a special file and locked with a password would simply disappear. This happened twice. Eugene finally found one of these songs after searching through some remote archive in the computer; the other has still never been found. Sometimes when we had laid down a good vocal we would begin the next day only to find the recording completely garbled, and we would have to rerecord it. Eventually, to circumvent problems, we would have backups of backups of backups, but the tricksters would always find other ways to challenge us.

Spirit forces can easily mess with electronic equipment, and this play of light and dark soon became part of the digital software behavior. Fortunately this also worked to our advantage when spirit musicians would insinuate their own editing into our efforts and improve on them. Many were the times when one of us would say to the other, "We didn't put that in, but damn, it's good!" We never argued with these adjustments that were always for the better. On one occasion we did not like a particular ending to a song and deleted it, thinking the song would do better without it. The ancestors disagreed, and when we played it back in its new edited state the deleted music was still there even though the digital display of that section was not. Eugene and I gazed at each other in dismay while Eugene stated, "But Dave, that's just impossible, it can't happen!" We put the ending back again digitally where it belonged. From these escapades both of us learned much about how the spirit world can work electronically in the metaphors of Harry Potter and Lord of the Rings.

Kabbalah, *sangoma* and Celtic wisdom have a lot of light to shed on this subject. Our adventures with this play of light and dark in the recordings can be extrapolated to how the cosmic "Field" really works. Moreover, dark and light forces can meddle most easily with modern-day digital equipment, and it was in this arena we began to marvel at their respective expertise, even though we never enjoyed it when it came from the tricksters.

On one occasion Eugene had a dream in Hebrew stating, "hamaskil yavin," meaning, "the enlightened understand." We both realized from the outset that this music was for the select ones, mainly those under duress who needed healing. The melodies were also for meditation, guided imagery, and for dreaming. Several of my patients had much speedier recoveries from a surgery or a devastating illness by being able to listen to the songs on a device while in the hospital. Others have used them for self-healing or play them before going to bed at night for better dreaming. In the case of children, they can help prevent nightmares and give kids a more restful sleep. Eugene and I have joked that it is great music to die to, and I know of several people who, after being very agitated, became calm and peaceful before journeying over to the other side.

Most folks find the songs calming and relaxing, but are so accustomed to performances by top musicians and superb vocalists that they possibly get stuck in the roughness of the form instead of being able to find and feel the essence of the compositions and their "vibration."

VI

inception

"There is a dream, dreaming me." – Bushman saying.

*Listen with your heart, risk being a fool and
risk all if you would gain all.*

*Mind shapes and defines the heart.
Imagination creates possibilities, choice sets the intent,
and will activates and actualizes.*

AROUND THE TIME I BEGAN MY INITIATION TO BE A *SANGOMA*, I had an epic dream of an incredibly numinous and luminous African landscape. In the dream I was driving to my ancestor uncle Sam's farm and I arrived in a magical place. I was in a valley, and on one side of the valley was a huge cliff or mesa, with rocks and stones that looked like they were shimmering with light. There was also a ledge two-thirds of the way up the cliff leading to a further elevation up to the top of a dramatic cliff face that was quite flat. The ledge ran right across the length of the cliff. There were other less remarkable cliffs on the opposite side of the valley. Two Bushmen came out to greet me.

This was what Carl Jung would have called a "Big" dream. *Sangomas* might call it an instructional dream from the ancestors. This "dream place" presumably was where I was being told I could explore my *sangoma* potential to the full. It would be a special place to explore the use of medicinal plants, which component had been lacking in my initiation. It had always been my dream to have a place in the bush in South Africa, and this seemed to be confirming that this was in line with the ancestors' plans for my work.

After that vision I could not rest. I looked all over different parts of Limpopo in the far north of South Africa, where the dream seemed to have taken place, for the same rock topography and a similar mountain. It was first at a friend's farm called Lesheba that I began to look more closely at the magical Soutpansberg mountain range where I thought I might find this special mesa. After spending a lot of time in the Waterberg mountains and elsewhere in Limpopo province, I had drawn a blank, and I was now beginning to try to make anything that I could find fit my dream. Nothing, however, seemed to quite comply with the original vision.

In the late 1990s I spent a ten-day period on a solo retreat at Lesheba while the family had gone to the coast for Christmas. I spent the time walking the land and exploring the mountains. The fact that it was well stocked with game made it all the more enthralling. I became enchanted with this area called the Soutpansberg (Salt pan mountains). Lesheba was named after a mountain called Lesheba. The property, and the adjacent farm, Dundee, both shared Lesheba mountain. Dundee was for sale. Although the mountain did not quite fit with the vision of my dream, there were some similarities. However, Dundee was inundated with alien, invasive eucalyptus trees, which made the land feel foreign, dark and foreboding. Nothing grew in their shade. It stood in stark contrast to the pristine Lesheba, next door.

While I was there, I went to the top of a cliff overlooking Dundee and threw my divination bones to see if this was the right place for me. Lesheba mountain somewhat resembled my dream, although this needed a stretch of my imagination. The bones seemed to indicate a satisfactory, but not overly enthusiastic, endorsement. One of the bones, however, seemed to be pointing more to the farm to the east of Dundee, the one I was later to learn was called Uniondale.

I chose to ignore this at the time, and felt that the bones had endorsed the purchase of Dundee. I met with the owner, but his price was so outrageous and his attitude so adversarial and arrogant that I decided to go no further. Later on I was to have further trouble from this individual.

In May 2002, when I was back in California, I received a call informing me that Dundee had gone into foreclosure. The owner had managed to retain a small amount of land around the homestead when the bank had taken over the rest. He intended to continue using it as his personal retreat, while the broker planned to sell off the remainder. If I wanted to buy the farm, I could. I might have felt enthusiastic but for the eucalyptus trees, the price, the slight misgiving remaining after the mountain bone divination, and the prior meeting with its original owner.

The broker wanted my commitment immediately, otherwise he was going to sell it to somebody else. I told him I would call back the next day with my answer. The following day I called him with my promise and told him I would fly out shortly to complete the purchase. The price was still too high for my means, but it was much lower than the price I had been given when I had discussed it with the owner a few years earlier. I was hoping I might be able to turn the eucalyptus forest into lumber to offset the cost, and at the same time "purify" the land.

No sooner had I arrived in Johannesburg than I learned that the farm had been sold to a more "suitable" buyer! I was disappointed and angry with the broker because I had made the long trip only to negotiate the purchase. However, ultimately the outcome proved to be for the best.

Around that time, a friend of mine had visited a farm next to a game reserve called Medikwe. The farm was in the northwestern part of South Africa, bordering on the Kalahari Desert, quite close to the Botswana border. It is a magnificent "Big Five Reserve" with a plethora of game. He told me of an amazing opportunity on the border of the reserve. Apparently the Park Board's intention was to drop the fences on one side and incorporate the adjacent farms into the park. This meant they would then be traversed by big game. Medikwe's borders would be enlarged and the farmers would benefit at the same time, a win-win for all concerned. He said this would be a good time to get in before the prices escalated. The game rangers at Medikwe were aware of this development and knew of one of the local farmers who wanted to sell half of his farm bordering on the fence.

I decided I may as well go to Medikwe and check out this alternative offer. When I arrived and chatted with the game rangers they all confirmed this amazing opportunity. Although the area did not in any way fit with my dream, I was excited with this prospect, especially since, after all the searching, there seemed no other viable options.

I went to visit the farmer, saw the land, and had a long discussion with him about the quite ordinary 500 hectares of flat bush. The only compelling part of it was that it would be in big game country, hopefully within the year. The farmer was adamant that this was going to happen and explained that he did not need the extra land. He just wanted to retain the section that he was currently farming. The price was more affordable than Dundee and there was the added bonus of a large lake nearby with spectacular birdlife.

Three dreams antedated these events that are relevant to this part of the story.

Before I had left California, Maryellen had two dreams warning me to be careful. In the first, someone had come to her and said, "Tell Dave he must 'pas op for a *skelm.*'" This means he must be careful of a trickster or a con artist. A short while later, through a second dream, I was warned to be careful of a "*tsotsi,*" which is a gangster. Maryellen did not understand the meaning of either dream, which made it clear that it was not a projection of her sometimes overly protective psyche.

The one dream was already confirmed. The trickster broker had aborted my acquiring the Dundee property. I now wondered who the "gangster" might be, and also if it was this farmer.

I had a third dream around that time. I was "driving" in the tree-tops of the eucalyptus forest in Dundee in a 4x4 with a group. I told the group that I had spotted two leopards and drove toward them. As I got nearer I said, "No, they're not leopards, they're cheetahs." I drove yet closer until it was clear they were two baboons that had been painted with spots and made to look like cheetahs, with the emphasis on CHEAT! I had been "cheated" once already. Thanks to the three dreams I decided to research the truth of this Medikwe proposition further, in case I was now about to be conned by a second "cheetah" or the tsotsi.

I was lucky to get directly through to the official in charge of the local Parks Board. This is not always easy in South Africa. When I asked him about the possibility of them dropping the fences, he started to laugh. He told me that not only were they not going to drop the fences, but all those farms on that side of the park were under land claim and were soon going to be returned to their rightful owners! I thanked my ancestors for the dreams and drove back to Johannesburg.

I planned to go back to the Soutpansberg with Rupert Harris, a good friend, who is a tour director and who had been assisting me with my groups that I had been facilitating in Limpopo. He knew of a few other places for sale. He also recommended I speak to Ian Geiger, a prominent conservationist in the Soutpansberg. Ian would certainly know of any other land for sale. Ian was working with other farmers at the time to change the Soutpansberg Conservancy into a biosphere on the grounds that it was a unique ecosystem. Ian had a magnificent mountain retreat in the area called Lajuma and told me that he knew of someone who was selling his farm, Uniondale, just to the east of Dundee. Of note was the fact that the road to Dundee traversed the Uniondale property as an easement. The previous nasty owner of Dundee used this road to gain access to his homestead rather than go the much longer route around through Lesheba.

I recalled the prior bone reading and that the bones had possibly been pointing to this farm east of Dundee. Perhaps I had misconstrued the true message, since Uniondale had not been for sale at the time. I now realized I might have been barking up a eucalyptus tree on the wrong farm. I called the owner of Uniondale, who told me that George Sioga, his foreman, would show me around. The farm was affordable, and it was exactly where I wanted to be.

Rupert and I drove up a terrible 4x4 road in my newly acquired second-hand 4x4, 1987 Toyota. The road was pitted with potholes and had a challenging middelmannetjie (translated as "middle man," a raised ridge in the center of the dirt road) so prevalent in off-road South Africa. We arrived at the top of a truly spectacular place with a stunning view of the mountains to the north. After a frustrating 10 days, I did not even appreciate that the place fitted the topography of my "Big dream" in every detail! It was only some time later that I realized the mountains were the same. There was also a partially-built house on the property without any roof. The walls had been built by a gifted Venda stonemason, but there was no roof and no floor. There were only walls with some windows and doors.

I recalled that 15 years previously, in a shamanic ritual in the Amazon, I had experienced a dream-like vision of a house without a roof in a similar kind of valley in South Africa. The cliff, the ledge, the numinous and luminous rocks and stones of my more recent dream were not in the earlier vision in the Amazon, but the valley itself was similar, and this vision had also haunted my memory. I knew from my initiation that visions and dreams from the spirit world were not time bound and could be remembered when opportune. (This dream fits well into that category already mentioned, of dreams to "tend.")

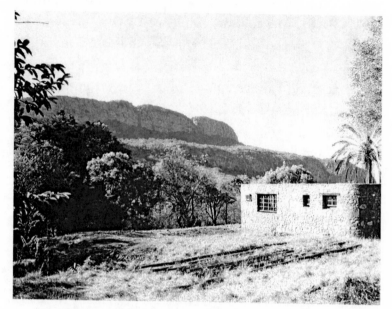

Mountain dream scape and the house with no roof

There were also a few interesting things that happened at the time of the visit which made me think it was meant to be. One was a delicate and graceful red duiker, an antelope, standing like a sentinel on the road close to the house just as we drove down to leave. George told us that on the way out we should visit a special riverine area with a pool. We went down to the spot where we found a magical glen with tropical over-growth and a pool with reeds, papyrus and a variety of indigenous subtropical plants. It was June, the middle of winter in South Africa. It was very cold, which made it unlikely that we would see any snakes. When we got to the bottom, lying in the grass close to the pool were two black mambas, about five to six feet in length. They were not moving on account of the cold.

At first I thought this might be a bad omen because the mamba is usually a warning in African tradition, but the two of them lying together in the grass and not moving seemed auspicious. The whole scene seemed very unusual and mystical, but I was concerned about conflicting messages. One was the beautiful red duiker and the other, the deadly, ominous mambas. In retrospect, the meaning was that both symbolic sightings were true, as I was later to find out. My ancestors were informing me that, though compelling, the land would also offer up many challenges and dangers. Free will allowed me to make my own decision about the purchase and undertaking, yes or no!

Andries, now my new *sangoma* mentor, lived in a town quite nearby, which was also serendipitous. Rupert and I took off down the mountain to see him and check out how it looked for the farm. When I asked him about the farm and the snakes his response was very simple. He said, "It means everything on the farm is alive and well. It's like if you go to a shop, all the things inside the shop are there, so if you want to buy it, it's good because all the supplies, all the things you need, are there for good business." His simple explanation gave me the all-clear to buy the place. The mambas and the duiker, he was saying, were a sign that the ecosystem was healthy.

In Polokwane, Rupert, the seller, the attorney and I sat down to sign the paperwork. I asked them whether there had ever been any land claims on the property and believed them when they said no.

Having purchased the farm, I left South Africa quite enchanted with the idea that I now had my place. This was July 2002. I was planning to come back in December of that year to start building, and in the meanwhile Rupert started to make inquiries about builders, roofers, and so on. Before leaving we went back to the farm to speak to George, who not only had building experience, but had been born on the mountain and knew the area intimately. He welcomed the opportunity to stay on, with a salary increase. There was a small house on the land where he was already living.

The first challenge was a defunct well, or borehole as it is called in South Africa, and an adequate water supply. Although the borehole had been operating in the past, there was no pump and we were unsure of the quality of the water. George needed to go down to the neighboring farm of Calitzdorp to get his water, which was several kilometers down the terrible road.

At that stage, I started to recognize some other signs that I had not realized before.

After the above-mentioned dreams of the farm I had been given two other dreams. During all these I was at ancestor uncle Sam's farm. Uniondale looked nothing like Sam's farm, which was 30 miles south of Johannesburg in the Highveld, but this did not matter in the dream. If anybody could have found me a place in the bush, it would have been Sam, who had been a farmer and African adventurer.

Sam was a colorful character, full of romantic stories of the old South Africa. As a youngster in his early teens, he had run away from home and illegally joined the army, lying about his age. After that he had gravitated to the diamond diggings, where he had been a boxer to make some extra money to make up for the lack of finding any diamonds. Sam was a tough character and an excellent marksman. As a boy he would enthrall me with tales of his experiences with the bad characters he met on his travels and how he outwitted them. His farm was my boyhood retreat where I could escape from Johannesburg to ride his horse, shoot and explore the then-virgin veld. I was present at the time he built his farm and watched him plan the design of his dream on the back of a cigarette box. In times to come I would feel that I was following in his footsteps in the building of *Tshisimane.*

I had one dream of a large baobab tree on Sam's farm, where, at 6000 feet of elevation, no baobabs grow. Baobabs are also not that common on the south side of the Soutpansberg – but one day as we drove up the road, George showed us a stunning baobab tree. The other dream was of a tall kipiersol or parasol tree. In front of the house on this land was a very tall, elegant kipiersol.

I now felt reassured that I had found the place of my dreams, and that the ancestors had sent me here. I headed back to California feeling satisfied that I had a 4x4 Toyota pickup, the land, a foreman and a defunct well. I would return soon to begin with the building.

VII

visioning
Tshisimane

THE JOURNEY TO INITIATION TOOK NEARLY THREE YEARS, and even after that I could best be compared to a neophyte doctor who had just completed his internship. Much was still required of me before I could become a competent *sangoma*. In a sense I was to complete the equivalent of a "residency program" at *Tshisimane* healing center. I would come and go there over the next several years from California for as long as three months at a time and at least twice a year.

The Soutpansberg mountains are situated about 100 miles south of the Limpopo River and the border with Zimbabwe. They straddle the main highway to the north, and run from west to east. The eastern part has a much higher rainfall, and hence is a lucrative farming area for subtropical fruits, much like Hawaii. The western side is very dry on the northern slope, and the rainfall on the southern slope is also quite meager. However, the southern slopes of the Soutpansberg, where *Tshisimane* was situated, are blessed by mist and fog that support a much richer plant diversity than their opposite side. This area also has spectacular cliffs, gorges, and valleys with thick subtropical bush. The whole area is well north of the Tropic of Capricorn.

In December 2002, at the time of a major solar eclipse in the northern part of South Africa, I returned to Uniondale to begin the process of building the healing center. I had invited Cecil, a boyhood friend of mine, a builder, to come and help. He lived abroad but was willing to come to South Africa to advise and assist me on the project. We arrived at the farm with some very basic camping equipment and enough food to see us through for a few days at a time. We needed to go down the mountain every now and again to replenish our supplies and buy building materials.

Faced with the prospect of a house without a roof, no floor, no toilet, no shower or any infrastructure whatsoever, we were nevertheless undaunted. We were buoyed by our optimism and our creativity. The thought of embarking on a new project lent a sense of adventure to our mission.

On the property there were the beginnings of a lapa, an area for sitting together, eating and meetings. Stones had been filled in between retaining walls so that folks could gather there to *braai* (barbecue) and enjoy the outdoors. This was a huge area with many animal skins from past hunting strewn about amongst the dirt and stone landfill between the walls. There was also an old goat shed with only two walls remaining where we planned to put the healing hut or *ndumba*. We began to envision what else was needed.

The history of Uniondale farm went back to the late nineteenth century when it was first purchased by a missionary, a Dutchman, called Bos. His gravestone was on the farm, together with several others. It seemed as if he, his children and his wife had all been buried there. Two of the graves were only large enough to be those of children. He had purchased the property in 1898, and some time later I uncovered a Deed of Sale to that effect that proved to be of significant importance. Bos died in 1923. His journey at Uniondale had been a difficult one, as evidenced by the New Testament reference on his tombstone:

> "I have fought the good fight, I have finished the course,
> I have kept the faith; in the future there is laid up for me
> the crown of righteousness, which the Lord, the righteous
> Judge, will award to me on that day; and not only to me,
> but also to all those who have loved His appearing."

My future house was going to be as rustic as possible, with as few conveniences as were necessary to live comfortably in the bush. My experience with the Bushmen of the Kalahari had taught me that the more things that you have, and the more you surround yourself with unnecessary "stuff," the less contact you will have with the elements and Mother Nature. This had the effect of diluting Her transformational and healing power. The intention was to maintain the walls of the house, which were beautifully constructed with local stone. A thatch roof was to be added, which was a challenge, because the house expanse was so large. There was a kitchen, a huge living and dining room, an outside area that was meant for a porch, one small bedroom, one huge master bedroom, a storeroom, a bathroom, and a separate toilet. These were separated by walls built on a raised landfill. There was, as yet, no concrete slab. The landfill dropped off to the garden below on the north side, where it was supported by a beautifully-constructed stone wall.

Unfortunately the Venda stonemason was nowhere to be found for further building. The owner at that time, who had been a retired policeman, had begun the task. He drank heavily and spent his time shooting the game on the property, hence all the dried-out animal skins. George told us that the policeman had attempted to cull the baboon troops as well. He did not pay his employees, and eventually ran out of money. The house had gone into default and the workers had left. He had been unable or unwilling to pay what was due to them.

The farm had been taken over by Leon Oosthuizen, who had sold it to me. He had owned it for only a short period before relocating to another farm higher up in the Soutpansberg. George, now my foreman, was born on the adjacent farm, Calitzdorp, and his father and grandfather had both been buried there. The missionary, Bos, who was the first white owner, had opened a school. Over the succeeding years there I met several people who had gone to that school and remembered the days when there was a thriving black community in the area led by a headman from the Matcheseve clan. Eventually he died and the rural folk moved out to seek jobs in the cities. There were very many good things that I learned about Bos and his school during my stay, and some of these events colored the local history on the Soutpansberg. Bos was a devout Christian who had done a lot of good for the Venda people living there at the time.

Venda huts are built of adobe reinforced with sticks. The roofs are made of thatch and the floors of cow dung. In a more modern but possibly less sophisticated way, the future homestead would follow similar building principles. The thick thatch, as well as the stone walls, would keep the inside cool in the hot summer months. Once it was built, I found that it could be more than 100 degrees outside, but inside the house was wonderfully cool, so much so that I would sometimes have to put on a shirt. However, the house was not as warm in the winter as it might have been if it had truly followed traditional lines with adobe and dung rather than concrete and stone.

the source

I renamed Uniondale "*Tshisimane*," which means "the source," "a spring," or can also refer to the Creator or the Source of all things.

The dirt road up to *Tshisimane* traversed the Calitzdorp farm below and went beyond Uniondale to the adjacent Dundee at the top. The new owners of Dundee proved to be wonderful neighbors who did a lot of land restoration and reintroduction of wildlife, though when I eventually left years later the alien eucalyptus groves remained mostly intact.

It was said that Jan Smuts, a former renowned Prime Minister of South Africa and founder of the League of Nations, had originally owned Dundee and had built the road. Apart from the main access that was the 4x4 dirt road up the mountain, there were some tracks that had been cut into the bush and up to the bottom of the mountain ridge, but these were overgrown. Over the next year we were to clear not only these, but a number of diverse trails over the roughly 1500 acres of scenic terrain. The road up to *Tshisimane*, with its red sand and challenging twists and turns, was labeled *bobbejaan* pad (baboon road) by one of our visitors who had at one time brought up a trailer full of furnishings such as tables and chairs for the house. Although he had carefully tied the load down, he unknowingly lost a number of pieces along the way. Fortunately I was driving behind him and managed to rescue those that had fallen off. The road was always challenging, even after attempts to grade it. Summer rains would make short work of these efforts. Though only eleven kilometers from the tar road, it would take 45 minutes to get up or down the baboon road.

VIII

Inward Bound

Remember the wisdom of wild things, the holiness of ele-
ments and the healing powers of waters.
Water trickling from the top of a hill
is but a drop of the deep spring within.

The breath that is in all beings emanates from the sacred
well spring making us all one – not the same but all one.

We should thank the stars for their song. Their light
emanates from their singing and when they sing they
glow. That is how they reveal themselves.
When we pray in the morning it is a
continuation of the singing of the stars.

The stars and the planets have a greater consciousness
even than that of humans and only slightly less than that
of the angels, as do stones, water, earth and air.

SOME YEARS EARLIER I HAD WRITTEN A BOOK ON THE HEALING
power of wild places called *Inner Passages, Outer Journeys.*
The travel company called Inward Bound became the experiential part of the book's philosophy. Through Inward Bound I
had been taking groups into remote pristine wilderness since

1995. These included places in California, Peru, the Sinai desert and Southern Africa, including the Kalahari. I very much wanted to extend the lessons from my Inward Bound philosophy to the building of *Tshisimane*. The fact that two Bushmen came out to meet me during my dream affirmed that what I had learned from the Bushmen on my many visits to the Kalahari should be incorporated into the plan. I intended to have the basic comforts for visitors coming to experience indigenous African healing, but knew I needed to keep as little as possible between them and the surrounding wildness for the most powerful spiritual effects. However, *Tshisimane's* design would need to include basic amenities such as beds or cots, good food, and hot water for showers.

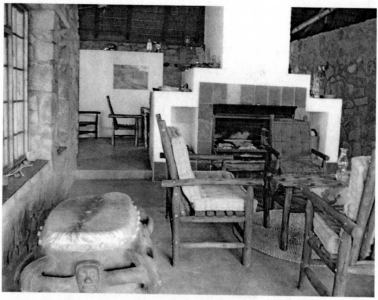

Living room and fireplace

Nature is a magnificent microcosmic representation of the Divine. Wilderness is God's showpiece. She is the ultimate healer and can afford the strongest medicine. Indigenous healers know this truth, and their "natural" medicine will never be outdated. Whatever is still wild and free is a powerful resource for healing.

I planned to embrace the concept of a Garden of Eden archetype at *Tshisimane*. It was a compelling wilderness area and I was committed to returning it as much as possible to its original pristine state. I knew that treks into some of the most remote areas on earth can be the best prescriptions for counteracting the burn-out of modern life, and that time spent in the wilderness can be one of the most powerful ways to promote well-being. This principle combined with ancient African healing wisdom seemed an ideal formula for total mind-body-spirit restoration.

Although most us may never attain the enlightened states of samadhi, or nirvana, we can experience episodes of bliss if we immerse ourselves in the wild outdoors in the right way. The untamed majesty of nature can induce what wilderness psychologists have called the "wilderness effect," which can be powerfully restorative. If one adds a spiritual component, it is not difficult to induce the more intense and transformational experience that I have called "Wilderness Rapture." This is somewhat similar to Maslow's idea of a peak experience. This concept of combining pure nature with ancient African "medicine" became part of the mission statement for the integrative healing that would occur at *Tshisimane*. Balancing the different polarities of left and right brain would help us access the feminine healing power in nature. If we were to restore ourselves deeply in the wilderness, we had to leave dominating, male, "left brain" ego and goal-oriented attitudes at home. A more intuitive, compassionate, feminine, "right brain" approach was required. I knew from my previous Inward Bound trips that no matter which it is – inner or outer directed, left or right brain, light or dark, feminine or masculine, sun or moon, yin or yang – we needed to balance the opposites to achieve wilderness rapture. When we focus only on physical pursuits, we lose the magic and the ability to heal and restore ourselves.

> To "achieve" is to be externally oriented, but to attain deeper effects we need to let go of the attachment to accomplish anything. Goal orientation and rapture are mutually exclusive in the present moment. We begin with a goal, but once the intention is set we should strive to detach from the possible outcome.
>
> David Cumes, M.D.
> *Inner Passages, Outer Journeys*

I knew this to be the crux between balancing inner and outer experiences.

The ability to be in harmony with oneself and with nature is embodied in the model of the Bushmen. Although they have largely lost access to their habitat and have almost disappeared as pure hunter-gatherers, their unique consciousness and their relationship with nature has always been an inspiration to me. The San Bushmen once inhabited the whole of Southern Africa, before the Bantu peoples arrived and encountered them there. I realized from them that nature alone could be one of the most powerful spiritual forces available for personal growth if accessed in the right way. If we simulated the Bushman model as much as possible, we could reconnect with that primeval hunter-gatherer part of ourselves which resides deep in our psyche. This is an intrinsic part of my own philosophy and also, I thought, the reason that the most powerful *sangomas* were usually found in intimate contact with nature. Even if, as Westerners, we do not have the skills to hunt and gather, we can at least keep it simple and connect with the land, the wildlife, the rhythms of nature and also the medicinal plants and edible foods that are so prolific in the bush.

The force of the primal self manifested as
love is the glory of God.
Those who awaken it in others and nurture
the nurturers glorify him.

The Bushmen reach higher dimensions of consciousness not by any esoteric practice, but by their intrinsic connection with nature alone and by exposure to the multifaceted properties that wilderness possesses. Their ability to transcend ego, open their hearts and travel out of body into the spirit world during their trance dance is a testament to this quality. The same is also true for the ancient *sangoma* paradigm, and this was what I wanted to access with the help of the older *sangomas* in the area.

The soul's language is learned by listening with the heart.
It has many sounds including that of silence.
Its eloquence is universal.

Wilderness is a natural and powerful catalyst for the inward journey and is diverse and varied enough to transform anyone who has the right intention. Nature herself can be a meditation, and solitude can be part of the experience. Wilderness is a "room with many doors and windows to spirit." The mantra of the bush, the sounds of the African night or of the wind or rain are all a meditation if realized as such. Furthermore there are constant fluxes in polarity to help one find balance and what Buddha called the "middle way." These polarities include up/down, light/dark, hot/cold, hungry/satisfied, terrified/tranquil, wet/dry, thirsty/satiated, etc. This realization helps one appreciate that experiencing nature's power is not always comfortable, but learning her ways is always rewarding, either literally or metaphorically.

*God's rivers of pleasure and good are not placid waters
of insipid purity. They have currents of all strengths,
frequently forking into wild twists and turns alongside
gentle flows, all churning and tumbling into swirling
pools too deep to fathom. They are for reflecting, playing
and rejuvenating, and then continuing
endlessly on to their source.*

If one added to this any number of inner-directed techniques such as meditation, yoga, breath work, drumming, chanting, ceremony and ritual, the power of the wild outdoors could be amplified tremendously. "Soft" fascinations occur in the space of sunsets, scenery, sights, sounds and smells. They seduce our senses and create enchantment and even rapture.

*"From my flesh shall I behold God." The route to God is
through our senses and is not to God but with God.*

On previous Inward Bound journeys I had discovered that many participants noted dramatic changes in the intensity of their dreams. There were also frequently major lifestyle shifts upon returning. Most called the trip one of the most significant events of their lives, so much so that there was frequently a profound reentry depression on their return that lasted several weeks.

I knew that for travelers who came to this remote part of South Africa, *Tshisimane* would offer an escape from the Western conditioning which influences so much of our behavior. Slowing down and focusing on essentials could free people from daily habits and patterns, opening horizons to new awareness. There was also a plethora of wilderness metaphors to connect with in the bush that could lead to further shifts in consciousness. In addition to the usual Inward Bound philosophy, daily dream and council circles, as well as divinations with the bones and healing rituals, magnified and actualized the power of nature. All of this provided a psycho-socio-spiritual milieu that could help the participants on their life journeys.

Balance is achieved by harmonizing polarities. Dualities come into harmony by negotiating a third or middle path, a path not of assimilation but of coexistence.

Solitude, furthermore, sometimes proved to be the most powerful of all catalysts, and often the more prolonged it was, the more illuminating was the experience. Select groups or individuals would do solo retreats in the multitude of suitable places that were available on the land to be totally alone with the fauna and flora. These "vision quests" had transformative spiritual effects on the seekers.

The most profound of all sounds is that of silence, not the silence that is the absence of noise, but that of the quietness in which we hear the longings of our heart and ponder our response.

Nature is an instrument for belittling the ego and disallowing it to dominate the Higher Self. This simple but profound connection with Her, the more austere the better, enables moments of enlightenment and personal revelation even for those who have difficulties with esoteric meditative techniques.

God's breath is heard in quietness and felt in stillness.
Beware the noises and clamor of ego which drown out the
Divine whisper.

In South Africa there tends to be an infatuation with the *"Big Five"*: lion, elephant, rhino, buffalo and leopard. Rupert, a naturalist who helped with the groups, was rather an expert in the "little five": the ant lion, the elephant shrew, the rhino beetle, the buffalo weaver, the leopard tortoise, as well as insects, butterflies, frogs and all the other creatures which were so prolific at *Tshisimane*. These little beings lent themselves well to an inner-directed experience and subdued the machismo that so easily surfaces in the African bush. The deeper one looked, the more wonder revealed itself. More knowledge did not make anything any less mysterious. We came to realize that ...

Sacred mystery is to be experienced, not to be deciphered;
to be entered, not to be decoded. Beholding all creation
with awe, one sees into its sacredness.

To me it also seemed that *"the deeper you go, the less you know,"* and this increased the sense of awe.

IX

construction

CECIL AND I GREW UP TOGETHER IN THE SUBURBS OF Johannesburg. We had retained our close friendship throughout the years. He thought nothing of leaving his home and family to come and help me with the project. We arrived at *Tshisimane* equipped with little more than the essentials we would need for an extended camping holiday. We set ourselves up a short distance away from the homestead on a plateau with a fabulous view of the mountains of my dream. We erected a rustic kitchen with a gas stove, a small gas fridge and a tarpaulin to protect the kitchen from the summer rains, and we slept in a tent. There were no ablution facilities. A cold shower consisted of a bucket with a spout at the bottom raised up on a rope slung over a branch of a mango tree. Other ablutions were done in the bush, bearing in mind the "leave no trace" techniques of bush camping. We were happy, filled with energy and in high spirits, content to be surrounded by the natural ambience of the bush and eagerly anticipating the creation of *Tshisimane*.

A major eclipse of the sun occurred in December 2002. The Soutpansberg and the surrounding area were peak viewing sites for observing the eclipse. Although it was a cloudy day, Cess and I waited and watched for the sky to clear so that we could witness this powerful event. The clouds cleared as the eclipse began, and we were treated to a glimpse of the moon as it moved across the sun. The sky darkened, the very air seemed to stand still, and the birds were quiet. Not a sound could be heard. It was as if nature herself was holding her breath. This took place at the same time that we began to construct *Tshisimane* and we felt it boded well for an auspicious start.

Rupert would come from time to time to socialize and assist us, and there were also a number of others who were very generous in giving their help. We had a variety of visitors popping in. This was no easy task, given the challenge of the road to the farm, so their support was much appreciated. One such friend arrived in the back of a *bakkie* (pickup) one evening, and as she overzealously hopped out, she disappeared down the side of the embankment alongside. It was dark and she had not seen the danger. We spent some time rescuing and recovering her. She was undaunted by her dramatic arrival and was a frequent visitor after that.

A landscape architect came for Christmas with a tasty Christmas pudding and helped us design the landscaping. A fellow from Louis Trichardt (now renamed Makhado), the local town, made the arduous drive up the formidable road to help us with the well, which had been essentially pumping mud. He told us that it needed to be drilled out and a new "sleeve" placed inside. He did not even charge for the visit. He had enjoyed the experience and the conversation. For him it was about meeting someone new, unusual and interesting. I came across this sort of camaraderie quite often in my time at *Tshisimane*. It reflects a generous aspect of South African hospitality where people are willing to go out of their way just for the sake of it. Eventually we would install a solar water pump to work the borehole. Until then, we drove down the mountain to Calitzdorp to fill our five-gallon containers. My *bakkie* became our workhorse and our transport.

George told me that his grandfather had been a *sangoma* and had been responsible for doing male initiations in the area some time ago. He seemed doubtful of my *sangoma* capacities but politely said nothing. He was an inscrutable man, a product of the old apartheid era, and he kept his opinions to himself. He was brought up under the domain of "white supremacy," and it was an intrinsic part of his relationship with white people to be deferential, though he was never defensive or subservient. George was not quite sure what to make of me, a white *sangoma* who was taking on a major construction project with not too much in the way of technological know-how.

My intention from the outset was to have solar and wind power, and we were fortunate to find an expert, Koos, in Polokwane who came out to give us an assessment of our power needs. Koos knew the best solar-powered water pump to work the well once it had been drilled and re- sleeved. The Grundfos pump was state of the art, and was powerful enough to pump the water up the hill to a holding tank on the top of an incline above the house. This afforded us enough water pressure. Of course there were many problems, trials and errors, as well as numerous changes.

The weather was very changeable. One could experience all seasons, sometimes in one day: mist, clouds, wind or rain, and then beating hot sun. Summers were hot, with balmy nights and not too much humidity. Winters were sunny and warm to hot in the daytime, but cold at night.

We installed a wind generator to make power when there was no sun, and it was serendipitous that usually when the sun failed due to the cloud cover, the wind would come up the canyon and move the generator propeller. On rare occasions when there was no sun or wind, we used a gasoline-powered generator to work the water pump and feed the house. This conveniently plugged into the back of the solar panel dedicated to the Grundfos pump. The generator could also be used for welding. This was the only time that the blissful silence and insect-animal-bird mantra of the bush was broken.

Andre, our builder from Polokwane, was a tough Afrikaner who still believed that he was living in the apartheid era, which is to say that his attitude toward the black workers was not always polite. He was short and squat, with legs like tree trunks, and he had the "beer belly" typical of those whose primary recreational activity is drinking beer and *braaing* boerewors. "Boerewors" are the farmers' sausages so beloved in South Africa. They are an essential ingredient in any barbecue or *braai*. Boerewors is usually made of pork and beef, and the more fat in it the better.

Andre did not take kindly to any man who questioned his authority, and his workers found him a formidable taskmaster. They were intimidated by his powerful manner. He was an angry, sullen man, intolerant and aggressive towards his black employees. In the true manner of those bred in the apartheid regime, he was less belligerent towards his fellow whites. He had a strong belief that he was invincible and he once took on a huge boulder that four of his laborers, working together, could not move. To his chagrin, he could not budge it either. The onlookers said nothing. They knew what would happen if they laughed. Andre arrived at *Tshisimane* one day riding a small red tractor that was not in any way up to the tasks at hand. Andre had no farming experience and George found the tractor hugely funny, but he, too, kept his amusement to himself. Unfortunately, in the northern part of South Africa, some old racist behavior still prevailed.

Willem, the roofer, also came from Polokwane and was of a similar disposition. According to him he was the best thatcher far and wide. He seemed competent to handle the technical challenges of the extensive expanse of thatch. He invited us to come and see some of the structures he had done elsewhere, which were quite impressive. Unfortunately, he proved not to be as competent as he bragged when it came to *Tshisimane*.

Like Andre, Willem loved the bush and was entirely at home with beer, *braai* and *boerewors*. He was a likable, tall, well-built fellow, also overweight and with a beer belly. He wore the universal uniform of that part of the world: khaki shorts, a short-sleeve shirt stretched over a protruding stomach, *veldskoen* (shoes made for the veld) and long socks pulled up to his knees. The only thing missing was the not uncommonly seen comb sticking out of the top of his socks. He was self-righteous and arrogant and, though friendly and polite, insisted that things be done his way. He was sure he was the right person for the challenge and would never acknowledge that he might possibly make mistakes. Subsequent events proved him wrong.

Cess, as my friend Cecil was usually called, being a builder was invaluable in forming the layout for the homestead and in helping purchase the basic supplies and equipment that we would need. It was clear from my dreams that a ritual bath was essential for healing people, and it would be medicinal as well, since medicinal plants were always added to ritual baths in *sangoma* medicine. The medicine dispensed would be appropriate for the condition that had been diagnosed with the bones. Cess was also in the swimming pool business, and he brought along some good ideas for the outdoor bath. We took to the job of making the bath, which we decided to put behind the old goat shed site where we proposed to build the *ndumba* or healing hut. Additional walls would be erected around the existing ones to complete the layout where there was already a clearing for concreting a floor. Later on it would be thatched, along with the lapa. The major construction of the house would begin after Christmas, after I had returned to California.

Cess and I went down to Makhado, bought a 1000-liter plastic water tank, and had it cut in half. We proposed to place it in the ground so that the bath would be waterproof. Later on this would be plastered to give it a nice finish. The digging of the hole was a challenge for us because there were huge rocks behind the goat shed that required digging and extracting with a crowbar, all done by hand. George and Andre's workers were otherwise occupied. Cess and I eventually managed to dig the hole and place the plastic drum inside of it. The water outlet for the bath was plumbed to feed the garden, but the final plumbing and heating would have to come at a later date.

Just as we were deciding we needed to take on extra help, a man came up the road looking for work. His name was Dennis. He claimed to be an expert on tree felling. He had brought along an old rusty chain saw that was precariously held together with wire. It appeared to be more hazardous than any of the serious dangers inherent in tree felling. Intrigued, Cess asked him how we could be sure he was as good at his job as he claimed to be. He scooted up a tall eucalyptus tree with alacrity and we gave him a job.

One of the things that had still to be done was the downing of the eucalyptus trees, which were sucking water from the water table. There is a well-known reaction in South Africa whenever there is any reference to these trees: "Do you know how many liters of water a eucalyptus tree can suck up in a day?" The answer could vary from 50 to 500 liters and even more! There was no doubt that our trees were sucking up the water table and making the well water a muddy, brown-red color. Ant nest infestation within the iron-laden well sand added to the disconcerting red color of the water. This iron content in the sand also colored the dirt roads an attractive red.

Half of these eucalyptus trees were around the homestead itself, and though planted in earlier times for shade and a windbreak, they were now parasitizing the ground water source. The rest of the eucalyptus trees were in a glade below the house. All were offensive to the eye, not fitting in with the subtle colors and ambience of the indigenous bush. There was also a scattering of jacaranda and guava trees which needed to come down because they also were invasive and alien. We planned that all the trees were to be indigenous except for a beautiful oak tree next to the house that afforded shade and some palms that had been planted around the house, giving it a tropical feel.

Bos, the missionary, had planted cedar trees around the gravesite, a ten-minute walk to the east. These certainly had to remain even though they looked uncomfortable and somewhat haggard in the tropical heat. Although we cleaned up the gravesite, this never lasted long because the baboons would come from time to time and turn the stones over to look for grubs and insects. We never managed to keep the gravesite in a decent condition because of the baboons.

Andre began initiating the project, grumbling incessantly about his workers. We proposed to put the storeroom, the generator, and the batteries for the solar and the wind pump next to an already existing corrugated iron dam above the house.

The panel for the solar pump would be close to the storeroom and the panels for the house would be on the roof of the storeroom. These working parts of the farm were on the south side above the house, and later an attractive fence of insect-resistant sisal poles was placed around them so that they could not be seen. The corrugated iron dam was painted a rich green to fit with the bush tones.

The dam, filled by the summer rains, was used for irrigating the garden. The water was full of frogs, insects, mosquitoes, even sometimes the occasional snake, and was not fit for drinking. The potable water was going to come from the well and the holding tank above the dam. The most gratifying thing about the construction was that nothing had to be submitted to any local council and no official drawings, permits or codes complied with. We could do whatever we wanted there. This reminded me of how my uncle Sam had designed his farm.

The solar panels and other key items were protected from theft by special medicines placed in strategically positioned baboon skulls found on the property. These proved effective, since when I returned later from California I learned from George that two men, intent on stealing solar panels, had walked up the eleven-kilometer dirt road to *Tshisimane*, bypassing my panels. They walked another several kilometers into Lesheba where they had dismantled several solar panels and carried them out—quite an energetic undertaking. They had left *Tshisimane*'s solar system alone.

An architect came by one day, brought by the owners of Lesheba. He sketched a rough plan for the house that included some excellent ideas on designing the available space, notably the huge living, dining and kitchen area. He partitioned the space intelligently with a chimney and fireplace between the living and dining areas that could warm them both and the kitchen at the same time during the cold winter nights. These were common at *Tshisimane*'s 3000-foot elevation.

By the time Cess left, the ritual bath was situated, Andre had begun to build, and Willem was on board for the roof. I stayed on a couple of weeks before leaving to be sure everything would go forward in my absence. Rupert was to be on hand for questions and we were to be in touch by phone and email. The house was going to be constructed first, followed by the lapa (the barbecue or entertainment area) which would be built simultaneously with the healing hut. At a later date the ritual bath would be completed, with another water tank and an outside furnace (or in local jargon, a "donkey") installed. A fire is built underneath the steel tank of the donkey, affording hot water for the bath.

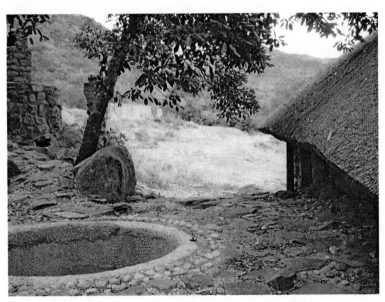

Ndumba and ritual bath when completed;
Sisal fence concealing the dam in the background

There remained only one thing to do before I left for California, which was to thank the ancestors for bringing me there and to initiate the inception of *Tshisimane*. I invited Andries to the farm with his three wives and several others. I went to pick them up and managed to squeeze them all into the *bakkie*, together with their drums and *sangoma* paraphernalia. George had helped me find a white goat and the plan was to make a sacrifice of the goat and have a ceremony and a ritual to invite the local spirits to support us at *Tshisimane* and thank our ancestors and guides for bringing us to this magnificent part of the world. The group disembarked from the *bakkie* with their drums and mats, and a suitable ritual with lots of drumming, dancing, eating and celebrating was offered with the goat to welcome the spirits. Goat meat, though a suitable offering for the ancestors, is very tough, but Andries and his huge extended family enjoyed the offering at home after the rituals were complete.

On this visit I was also fortunate in meeting Mabata, a fellow *sangoma* who had been a part of the African National Congress (ANC) that fought the war against apartheid. He had been a *sangoma* for the ANC guerrillas in the bush. He was enthralled with the idea of an indigenous healing center and very much wanted to be involved. It was he who suggested the name "*Tshisimane*" for the center. We both liked the idea of a *sangoma* museum and I proposed to start collecting *sangoma* artifacts from the local tribes. He was convinced he could obtain support at a governmental level for the project and even have the terrible road upgraded. We began our relationship, and friendship, with me performing a divination for him. It was clear that he was somewhat concerned about his own safety. I noticed that before the divination he removed a pistol from his pocket and placed it outside the sacred space where the divination was performed. At a later date he asked me, "Did you know that duiker brains are very good for protection?" When I explained that there was not going to be any hunting or harming of animals at *Tshisimane* I could see he was disappointed. He seemed worried for himself.

It was with a lighthearted, good feeling that I left *Tshisimane* and headed back home with the knowledge that, hopefully, everything was going to be under control with all the people that had been brought into play. In spite of all the precautions, however, I was to find there would be significant challenges.

I was fortunate that a good friend, Chris, spent several weeks at *Tshisimane* in the five month gap that I was not there. Chris had come with me to Limpopo some years back with a group on an Inward Bound trip. He had had a "shade," or intrusive spirit, over him at that time and we had laid it to rest on the trip. On that journey he became very enamored with South Africa. When he heard about *Tshisimane* he volunteered to spend time there, doing a personal vision quest and renewing his connection with the bush. Chris played a vital role in monitoring the building. During that critical time when I was not there, and when the roof was being constructed, he was able to oversee and recognize deficiencies in the work. Whenever he was very concerned he would report the faults to me.

It appeared that Willem tried to take shortcuts. All the wood poles and thatch had to be hauled up the horrendous road to the top of the mountain tied down to the roof rack of a 4x4. Since I was not there, Willem decided to make life easier for himself by skimping on supportive poles and concrete. His egocentricity and misplaced over-confidence led him to believe he could pretty much get away with anything and still do an acceptable enough job. Fortunately Chris was on hand to relay this information to me.

Chris reported that the roof was extremely heavy because of the vast expanse of thatch that covered the entire building, and that the weight could not safely be supported by the poles that had been used. In fact, when they had removed the scaffolding supports after thatching the roof, the roof had collapsed and Willem had to jack up the structure so that it could be patched and reinforced. Chris was unhappy about this and suggested that I bring in an engineer to confirm his fear that much more reinforcement was needed. Willem, in his arrogance, believed that there was no one who could second-guess his expertise. The engineer we consulted to review the situation initially confirmed that the roof supports were sadly deficient. Willem, however, was so forceful that the engineer was intimidated into making compromises with his original recommendations.

Yet another problem was to prove even more challenging. Because Willem was in a hurry, he decided to complete the roof before the chimney for the fireplace had been built, which had not been part of the original plan. The chimney would have further supported the heavy thatch. Willem was behind on his other work schedule and would not wait for Andre's chimney to be finished. Hence once the roof was completed, Andre had to cut a hole in the thatch to allow the chimney to come through. However, he now could no longer bolt the roof supports to the chimney. Willem argued that Andre was at fault for being tardy and keeping him waiting, and Andre correctly countered that Willem was impatient and negligent for going ahead prematurely. The result was a defective roof that, though patched from time to time, leaked during all the years at *Tshisimane*. Willem assured me that we were going to be "friends" for a long time and I was beginning to see why. There was a five-year guarantee on the roof.

In addition to the roof of the house, Willem had constructed a roof over the lapa. There were no complaints about this, although the poles were splitting, and were of inferior quality. Later we had to wire them with strong baling wire to prevent them cracking further. The roof of the lapa was a simple task and afforded a rain-proof structure without walls, meant for outdoor entertainment where we could *braai*, meet with people, do yoga, and have extra guests sleep over in the summer.

The *ndumba*, or healing hut, was another matter. The old goat shed still had two original stone walls standing. These walls had been made without any foundation or mortar. Willem decided these were enough to hold the weight of the roof on those sides and planned to use them instead of pole supports. Chris immediately recognized the folly of this and managed to coerce Willem to use poles instead. If not for Chris there would have been another problem down the road.

When I arrived in May 2003, the house roof looked adequate but the ridgeline was slightly concave where the collapse had occurred. The chimney flashing would prove to be a constant source of leakage from the rains. The lapa and *ndumba* were fine. Instead of going to the nearby riverbed, Andre had undercut the foundation on the north side of the house to get sand to mix into the concrete for the floor of the house. This undermined the foundation of the house, which was to prove a problem later when some of the walls began to shift slightly and crack. It also detracted from the aesthetics of the original plan. Andre had put up a makeshift stone wall where previously there had been a strong, attractive "Venda" wall. Andre's wall became a problem later when the heavy rains made it collapse, requiring reconstruction. Having spent some time in Peru, and being fascinated with the Inca stone technology, I reset the stones as I had seen them done there, and the wall held, after previous attempts by the workers to repair it had failed.

This visit coincided with that of a small group of women from Johannesburg, who had come for the first Inward Bound indigenous healing experience at *Tshisimane*. There were many building corrections that had to be made and fortunately, one of the members of the group, Trixie, was not only an expert at managing properties but seemed to have both legal and building expertise. I arranged for her to supervise and help sort out the challenges when I left, since Chris had already returned to the USA. Trixie, who lived in Johannesburg, would come out from time to time with her lawyer husband, Hennie, to check on the work. She made sure that Willem would attend to the roof, and Andre would see to the outstanding house issues. All difficulties appeared solvable since Trixie was a tough, no-nonsense lady who was more that a match for Willem and Andre.

While I was there, we undertook to remove the eucalyptus trees and managed to solicit a tree expert called Bernie. Bernie was not only tall, good-looking, tough and intelligent, but was also a pleasure to work with. He was full of good advice. On his first visit he came up the mountain on his off-road motor bike, but later came in with a crew. In no time at all the huge hundred-year-old blue gums were safely down, which made a big difference to the well water. This took some skill, since the house could have been demolished if he miscalculated the fall of a tree. Some lumber colleagues of his offered to remove the huge amounts of lumber if they could come up with their new portable, Australian-designed planking machine which would cut up the lumber on site. We assumed it would be ideal for the Aussie eucalyptus. They would then truck out the planks and remove all the extra wood that cluttered up the site, gratis. However, this idea to clear the area had to be abandoned since, when they began to cut planks, they found the wood to be of inferior quality. I was told this was because of a fire that had affected the wood grain many years previously. Our solution was to cut them up into circles that we used for paths, and later for a labyrinth.

The well now had a new sleeve and casing. The water pump was pumping delicious, pure, clear water for the first time. The solar was operational with the panels affixed to the roof of the storeroom which also housed the batteries, tools, chain saws and other farming essentials. The solar lights in the house worked, and an energy-efficient fridge was installed. Koos, who had arranged and installed all our energy requirements – solar, wind, and generator – brought in a six-burner gas stove and oven so that we were able to entertain sizable groups. It remained only to equip an effective kitchen, and that was done on a subsequent visit with the help of female expertise. The house still lacked furniture and cupboard space, but *Tshisimane* was beginning to take shape.

When Andre eventually completed his part of the building, Trixie reconciled the account with him, making sure that we did not pay the full price for his shoddy work. He did not seem to object to the discounted price on his original quote.

Everyone who came to *Tshisimane* was enchanted with the aesthetics and beauty of the place. It seemed that only George, Rupert and I were somewhat jaded by our experience of what had happened. At the end of the day, I had to admit that the fact that the construction had been successfully completed was somewhat of a miracle, considering the challenges and hardships of building on top of a mountain with extremely poor access and limited funds. Although I was sometimes frustrated by its blemishes, it was still fine for the work I was to do in the limited time available. I looked at the building saga not only as a lesson in non-attachment to the material world, but also as a tribute to the power of polarity balance that embraced so much of Inward Bound's nature philosophy. It was in the play of the opposites that one found balance, between light and dark, good and bad, efficient and inefficient, competent and incompetent, honest and dishonest. I recognized that in this "flux," sufficiency prevailed in spite of many imperfections. I was grateful to Andre and Willem for their expertise and work, and more especially to all the workers, most of whose names I never even knew.

All allies are not friends nor are all antagonists enemies.

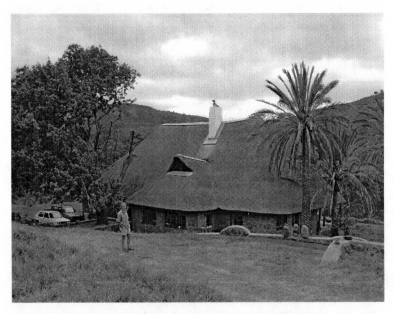

Lodge with the infamous chimney and flashing

Before I left for California, I decided to get hold of Gladwyn, who had introduced me to Mabata, because I was having
difficulty in contacting him by cell phone. The concept of a
healing center run by a white doctor and *sangoma* had been
especially intriguing to him and he wanted to support it with
his powerful connections. After numerous failed calls to him, I
drove to Makhado to visit with Gladwyn and inquire further.
Gladwyn was an herbalist working in the town. Though an
"herbalist" to any Westerner, she dreamed the plants she used
for her clients and was closely connected to the ancestors. I sat
down with her over a cup of tea and asked her about Mabata.
I was shocked to hear that he had died. I was interested in the
circumstances, but she was evasive and only said that he had
been sick and his kidneys had failed, which seemed surprising
considering how young and robust he had been when I last saw
him. She seemed reluctant to give me any further information.
I recalled his earlier security concerns and knew that Mabata
had been running for a local *sangoma* election. She told me
that another candidate who was running at the time for the
same position had also mysteriously died. I asked her if he had
been poisoned, but she just shrugged her shoulders. It is for-
bidden to accuse anyone of witchcraft, sorcery or being a witch
in Venda, so I understood her reluctance to say what may have
really happened.

Venda is renowned for its history of poisonings, and this
diabolical practice exists there even today. Chiefs and kings
were known to have their own personal cook and taster for
good reason. I had even been told that when drinking from
a vessel or gourd that had been tasted and tested, it was still
prudent to be sure that you drank from exactly the same area
that had touched the taster's lips, since poison could have been

impregnated on the opposite lip of the vessel offered without the brew itself being tainted. George told me some time later that when land claims were lodged and an adversarial relationship developed between him and the claimants, after that he would never eat or drink if he was invited to talk to any of them. There are numerous highly poisonous plants indigenous to Venda, unknown to Western science, that would never show up on a toxicology screen. I tried to explore this further with regard to Mabata's family. I called a few times, but got nowhere and decided to let the matter rest. I was extremely upset about this unhappy event.

I later became familiar with some of the trees that were traditionally used for poisoning. How they are prepared remains a secret, the province of witches and sorcerers, who will orchestrate such nefarious deeds for a hefty fee.

These poisons were also used in days of old as ordeal poisons—the ultimate lie detector test—to determine if someone was guilty of a crime, such as murder. The accused was given the poison to drink on the basis that if he was guilty he would perish, and if not he would vomit it up and survive. There is a possible medical explanation for this based on the faith of the innocent and the guilt of the perpetrator. An innocent person, trusting in the ancestors, would probably reflexively vomit up the vile-tasting potion. The terrified guilty party, on the other hand, would likely have a massive discharge from his sympathetic nervous system, as well as a high concentration of adrenalin circulating in the bloodstream. This would make the intestinal tract relax and be far more receptive to the toxin. Hence the poison would be rapidly and lethally absorbed. Presumably indigenous wisdom over the years had found this to be reliable and fair justice. No doubt the *sangoma* presiding also would have divined before the test to ensure that the party was in fact most likely guilty.

Kahuna shamans of Hawaii were known to have a similar way of administering justice. They would simply curse the guilty party, knowing that guilt plus an effective curse was as sure as a death sentence. Guilt has a profound effect on a person's ability to overcome psycho-spiritual obstacles, and if at a deep psychic level one believes one deserves to die or be punished, with the help of these techniques they will probably succumb.

Many of us who grew up in South Africa knew of at least one instance of a healthy, usually male individual, who came to his employer and told him he was going home to die. The employer would take him to a physician, who would do a full work-up only to reveal nothing wrong at all. Nevertheless, weeks later the employer would learn that the person in question had in fact died. The combination of a curse plus guilt facilitates the power of any curse exponentially. These individuals at some level, conscious or subconscious, believed they had done something seriously wrong and probably believed they deserved to perish.

By the time I again left to go back to California, *Tshisimane's* infrastructure was reasonably intact. The ritual bath was lying dormant for the moment and was to be finished on my next visits, together with the landscaping and planting of medicinal trees and plants around the homestead. To facilitate all of this as well as the building of an outside double bathroom, we needed to buy a tractor and a trailer. From this stage onwards most of the building was going to be done by George and the staff.

Dennis was beginning to show signs of a drinking problem

and I signed on a third worker called Ralph, who had previously worked on the lower farm of Calitzdorp. I spoke to Bernie and he said that I should go down to Levubu and speak to Henry about a tractor. I took George down to Henry's huge tractor establishment. Levubu is an amazing farming area in the eastern Soutpansberg. Due to the weather it is perfect for the cultivation of mangos, macadamias, bananas, papayas and other tropical fruits. I liked Henry immediately. He was honest and forthcoming and showed us the tractor that he recommended and a huge trailer which could carry a sizable load of stone or sand for the walls that needed to be constructed. Henry assured me that although it was an old reconditioned Ford, it was much better than the newer Massey Ferguson 4x4 tractors that were more expensive, slower and not as powerful. This proved to be true, since around the same time my neighbor bought a Massey that gave him no end of trouble and required numerous reparative visits out to his farm. The old rebuilt Ford had no trouble going up and down the mountain except with a heavy load during rainy season when the road was very muddy. When I left, George had a tractor and trailer to proceed with the work.

I would return to *Tshisimane* frequently, and this afforded ample opportunity to complete the whole project. George proved to be expert in doing stonework. The fact that he had worked with the stonemason who had done the original stone walls helped his skills. The tractor and trailer were critical for the building, as it now became easy to cart loads of river sand and the necessary stones up the mountain for the job. I constantly hauled cement and other supplies from Makhado to feed the work. Over the period of the next couple of years we completed the ritual bath, paved the surrounding area, put in a "donkey" (the rustic wood burner for heating water), plastered the inner part of the bath and lined it with beautiful local pebbles, and also completed an outside double bathroom. The results at the end of the day were extremely gratifying.

X

wildlife, walks and wilderness rapture

The four beings of nature are the still beings, the growing beings, the wild beings and the talking beings. The still beings are of the earth element and are the stones, the earth. The growing beings are from the water element and are plants, grasses. The wild beings are from the air element and are animals, birds and fish, and the talking beings are from the fire element and are us. We are all connected, some of all in each.

Fire gave birth to light, water gave birth to darkness, the wind gave birth to spirit and earth gave birth to humanity. They are the four bodies which are the foundation of all creation beneath the firmament. All four "beings," still, sprouting, wild and human are composed from these four foundations and all these beings each have an angel that watches over them.

To experience the still beings you must touch them, to experience the sprouting beings you must listen to them, to experience the wild beings you must dance with them and to experience the human beings you must feel with them.

THE FARMS OF OUR EASTERN AND NORTHERN NEIGHBORS were well stocked with game, excluding the large predators like lion, cheetah and spotted hyena, and larger game such as buffalo and elephant. Most of the neighboring farms, however, had not been stocked, and this included *Tshisimane*.

The concentration of leopard in the Soutpansberg is possibly higher than anywhere else in Africa, and the other smaller cats such as caracal and wild cat are also present. There were frequent leopard sightings at *Tshisimane*, notably one huge leopard whose territory included the house.

Although the leopard did not present itself early on in my stay, it became more frequently heard than seen around the lodgings. The first time I saw him was driving up the road at night with a group. We saw a large leopard crossing the road some twenty yards in the distance. There was not enough time to get his details but later on his size was confirmed by Willem, who in the middle of the day saw it crossing the road. He said it was as big as a lion. The huge size of the cat was established by George one night when he was driving back up the road to *Tshisimane*. He saw a massive leopard at the side of the road staring at him. He hurriedly closed his window and drove on, somewhat intimidated. On another occasion a group of us were in the healing hut when the leopard walked right by us in the middle of the day. All we got was a glimpse and a growl, but everyone was thrilled. When we located the spoor we were impressed by the size.

One night a guest decided to sleep outside. I was worried about him sleeping too far away from the house. Because of the leopard I suggested he sleep on the porch, which was safer. He compromised by sleeping nearby, as he wanted to be under the stars. He awoke at midnight to see a large cat crossing the road below. He picked up his bedroll and went inside. The next morning, when we checked the spoor, it was apparent that the huge leopard had visited that night. The guest had slept very well. His mother spent a sleepless night worrying about her son being devoured by a large cat. She had said to me that night, "If he gets eaten I am going to kill you!" She had already lost one son, so the threat may not have been an idle one.

During my stay I began to look forward to the leopard calling at night close to my window. The perimeter of the house and the window of my bedroom were now included in his nightly patrols. Every few nights I would hear the characteristic leopard sound, like somebody sawing a log. I regarded this visit as a gift, as good as any special dream. On occasion when I would arouse myself and get out of bed and go to the window to see if I could spot him he was already gone or not visible in the dark. The leopard became part of the daily activity. Frequently we would hear the baboons or monkeys screeching nearby or in the distance, and we knew the leopard was hunting. From time to time we would come across baboon skulls and bushbuck remains, testifying to his hunting prowess.

There was also a leopard that periodically killed the cattle at Calitzdorp. I only saw this leopard once. It walked across the road one morning when I was en route to Makhado. It stopped on the other side behind a thorn tree and watched me for a few minutes before disappearing into the bush. This one was normal size.

For the rest, the smaller cats were more nocturnal and not frequently seen. On one occasion, however, I was lucky enough to see an African wild cat in the middle of the day walking down one of the paths. I also had a similar unusual daylight sighting of a large porcupine close up.

It's important to understand that game sightings while on foot, no matter how rich the fauna, are actually quite rare. When animals smell our human scent their flight or fight response kicks in and they take off. This is quite different from being in a game park where one's scent is hidden by the exhaust of vehicles. Also those creatures are habituated to cars and the humans inside them.

Perhaps the most unusual sight of all was on one of my daily hikes. On this occasion I had come out of the bush and joined the dirt road that led back to the house. I saw a long line of caterpillars head to tail following a silk thread across the road. The end of this procession could be seen in the bush behind and the head was well into the bush on the opposite side. To add to the spectacle they were all brightly colored. It reminded me of a joke we had as kids about "Why did the chicken cross the road?" In this case the answer for the caterpillars also seemed to apply – "To get to the other side!" It was the only explanation I had for this mysterious form of cooperation.

The baboons were prolific. There were a number of troops, not only around the upper farm but also a large troop down at the lower farm that had previously monopolized the macadamias. Frequently they would come around the house, especially when we were not there, and sit on the table and chairs on the veranda, often leaving their deposits along the way. When summer would come, even before the mango crop was ripe, the baboon troop would come through like a cyclone. Afterward there would not be a single mango to be seen, only leaves and broken branches scattered all about. George told me how a baboon had managed to enter the house one time when I was away. He had come into the house to find the baboon sitting on the kitchen table, and there was pandemonium before the baboon escaped in terror, having left its excrement all over the kitchen as payment for entry. It took George hours to clean up.

We had numerous Amaryllis plants (*gifbol* or Bushman's poison bulb) planted around the homestead for spiritual protection. These hallucinogenic bulbs are highly toxic and are lethal if eaten. It is only safe to use the bulb topically for wounds. On one occasion I watched a baboon next to the house uproot and devour an entire bulb. While munching away slowly he appeared unperturbed. It is said that if one is lost in the bush with no food that one can safely eat anything that a baboon consumes to ensure survival. I listened all the rest of that day for the possible sounds of a baboon tripping out on the psychedelic effects of gifbol but heard none. I walked in the bush and also asked George to look out for a baboon corpse but he found none. I assume, from this, that it really is not safe for humans to consume everything that the baboons can eat.

There were vervet and samango monkeys playing constantly in the surrounding trees. Watching them or the baboons always made for a very pleasant distraction when one was bored. Once I was lucky enough to be in the house when the baboons must have thought I was gone because George had taken the 4x4. They came around the windows, looking in, trying to enter and not being able to see me because of their own reflection in the glass. When I suddenly became visible they scampered off barking in a panic.

At times we would get warthogs grazing the freshly cut grass around the house. The bush pigs were prolific but tended to be shy and were usually not seen, but we always saw signs of their scat and their diggings. They are thought to represent the ancestors and also represent medicine, since they are always digging for roots and seem to know what is good to eat and what is not. Some *sangomas* pay great attention to which roots the bush pigs dig up and these sometimes feature among the *muti*s they use. When in my early explorations, having never seen a bush pig, I asked a game ranger what one looked like, his description was simple and graphic: "A bloody huge pig!"

Now and again we were gifted with sighting a huge Kudu bull with magnificent horns that would make an appearance through the bush. Red duiker were very prevalent, especially around the house, where they would come at night to drink from the different ponds where water collected. Bushbuck were the most plentiful of all the antelope. The delicate and agile klipspringers (Afrikaans for rock jumper) were frequently seen in the stony mountain outcrops.

Certainly with each visit there was always a reward, either in the form of stunning insects, incredible birds or unusual animal or raptor sightings, depending on the time of year.

There was an abundance of animal sounds at night. The bush babies or nagapies were especially intriguing, their call being very much like a human baby crying or being strangled – an eerie sound. At night, with the help of a powerful spotlight, you could see the glow of their huge eyes high up in the trees. On rare occasions I also saw them sleeping there during the day.

Birdlife was prolific. Black eagles circled frequently. There was a Cape vulture colony nearby and every now and then we were greeted by the sighting of a Marshall or a Crown Eagle. Purple Crested Louries were magnificent and there was an occasional glimpse of the rare Narina Trogon. My favorites were the crested guinea fowl with their clucking sounds that were ubiquitous wherever one hiked. All in all, the ecosystem was fairly intact and there were all kinds of brightly colored grasshoppers and varieties of butterflies and caterpillars.

Rupert was an expert in spiders and was always finding and picking up something to fascinate us. The moths flying around the house lights at night were sometimes as large as small birds. Snakes were plentiful, especially black mambas and spitting cobras. Pythons were more rarely seen, but one time when I was away a python down at Calitzdorp devoured Richard's midsized dog. George had previously told me about a huge python that frequented the pools around Calitzdorp.

When I was alone at *Tshisimane*, I would have more time for my yoga practice and would also hike regularly. This was when I connected with the fauna and flora in the deepest way. At other times I would hike with Rupert, George or other friends who visited, and of course a hike was always a part of the daily activity for groups that came. There were numerous options to choose from. There were easy hikes that paralleled our access road and would join with it intermittently. Most of this terrain was punctuated by spectacular trees, most notably several varieties of wild fig. There was one gigantic bush fig, which must have been several hundred years old.

Concerning plants and trees, do not overlook the splendor of their starkness; the drab and leafless have their beauty and their purpose too.

There is not a single blade of grass that is born of the earth that does not carry within her immense wisdom and immense heavenly power. Humility and awe let one see most clearly and hear most truly.

From the beginning of creation trees have conversed with one another and with all living things.

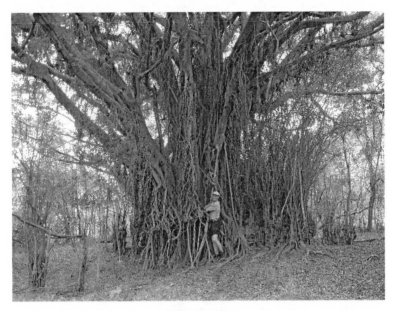

The Big Fig

There were other trees, such as Marula, Kiaat, Syringa, Boerbean, Moepel, Cape Ash and varieties of Acacia that were not only beautiful, but also medicinal.

To reach the northern mountain ridge that demarcated our property line from Lesheba, one had to climb an old 4x4 track. It was a short, though strenuous, climb to get to the lower ridge, where there were numerous spectacular vista spots. From here one could look down the valley to the south and to the east with views of Dundee to the west. One could then traverse the ridge, unless one chose to climb up to the top of the crest and walk along it. On one occasion, after doing this, I walked for about five hours with a guest all the way to Lesheba to visit our friends, who were kind enough to give us a ride back. After battling to get through areas of Acacia with their formidable thorns, we were not looking forward to a return hike of similar duration and bloodiness.

Another access path to the ridge climbed a spectacular but somewhat sketchy trail with some stunning flat rocks where one could sit and meditate at the top. Then one could make a loop and come back along the ridge and down the 4x4 track to the homestead. The flat areas on top provided perfect solitude for those who wanted to meditate. My daughter Romi did a four-day vision quest there, which brought back nostalgia for me when I would hike by from time to time after she had left. One of my tough Afrikaner friends was suitably impressed. I knew it by his statement, "Hell, man, you let your daughter be alone up there amongst the mambas, baboons and leopards for three nights?" Actually, Romi and other vision questers slept in tents at night, which ensured their safety from animals.

Hiking to the south of the house, one could climb up to a ridge which looked down precipitously onto the Vivo-Makhado road below and onto a flat, featureless bush-covered plain with the silhouette of the Blouberg mountain range to the west. There was also a spectacular deep gorge ten minutes walk south of the house that demarcated our boundary with Dundee. This was the baboon troop's favored spot and it was rife with baboon droppings. It very much had a "Lord of the Rings" type of magical appearance.

These hikes were among my best times at *Tshisimane*, when I would wander to my heart's content and enjoy whatever it was that nature presented that day. It was even more special during the summer thunderstorms when the rain would pour down, refreshing everything and rinsing one off from the heat of the day. On occasions, when lightning got a bit too close, the thunder would create cacophonies up and down the valley. Once I experienced a St. Elmo's fire-like effect when my hair stood on end due to the high voltage present between the clouds and the ground below my feet. Fortunately I was not vaporized.

Even now, some years after leaving, I have nostalgic dreams of the land and the wilderness rapture it so often provided. Andries had been correct with his reading in June 2002; the ecosystem was largely intact, with "a well-stocked shop of plants and wildlife." Moreover, it became my sanctuary and my temple, a continual source of renewal and replenishment. It was as if, when I hiked, the wilderness was actually meditating and healing me. Much of the time, even if I was not quite in a state of "wilderness rapture," I was in a state of deep inner peace. There was no doubt that I was being cleansed, purified and made whole while exploring the "four directions."

We are wrapped in the embrace of the winds, the mystery of the north wind, the inspiration of the east, the clarity of the south and the wholeness of the west.

The ancestors emphasize that words are important, but that they cannot tell all. We were instructed to ...

learn from the stones, the trees, the meadows and the waters, the air and the earth and every creature.

The ancestors also pointed out that the writings in my first book, Inner Passages, Outer Journeys, were expressing the early druidic "inner-scape of soul and outer-scape of nature" enabling one to see beyond ordinary reality into the magic of all things.

It is the sanctity of surrender that empowers the ability of the Higher Self to see the sacred in all creation. One can

see it in a pebble, a leaf or a feather, and also probe into
the uniqueness of all within the whole – endless diversity
in endless oneness. Surrender allows the inner Self to
silence speech so that we can hear the spirit voices of trees
and listen to the song in the winds. God's voice is heard
with the heart in response to its yearnings.

Indeed, nature-induced rapture can be found wherever one is. We can hear it in the sound of rain, feel it in a fallen feather, and see it in a spider's web. We need to consider everyday wonders that are unheard-of and overlooked, and which seem far remote from wilderness. This is sometimes called the "magic of the ordinary." With the right perception, even the smallest bit of the wild is capable of connecting us to our deeper Selves.

Converse with mountains, hills and valleys, with trees
and grasses, with crawling, flying and walking creatures,
with the planets and the stars and with
all manner of spirits.

The Celtic ancestors stressed how ancient druids exulted in the natural world because they saw it as a manifestation of the Divine. They knew that "stones and trees taught what could not be heard from the masters of words, much less the idle prattle of the ego."

An increased awareness of our natural connection with
rocks, trees, plants, animals – all the still beings, the growing
beings and the wild beings, not just the speaking beings –
is transformative. It will help us feel the special kinship
we have with earth, air, water, fire, sun, moon and stars

*and the sacred oneness of creation. This acknowledgment is
the beginning language of the realm of the non-ordinary. It
is the tongue of the spirit of all beings. If we are to
communicate with their consciousness we must learn
well this language of the senses.*

For myself, I became increasingly aware of the life force
in all the "growing things and the wild beings" and how all of
them were animated by the breath of the Creator. I was even
more aware of it when there were many, all interacting together. The chi or prana or ruach (Hebrew) or moya (Zulu) of the
plants, evidence of the Great Spirit's breath within them, was
sometimes quite palpable. As I walked I felt that the plants
were communicating with me in the way they best knew how
– maybe not personally to me, but generally as they would if
anyone was "listening." They were being all they could be even
in the most adverse of circumstances, when struggling to grow
out of a rock or survive submerged in a pool of water.

The ancestors also talk of the soft, still or silent voice of
God. For me that small voice within is sometimes heard as
conscience and sometimes as intuition. No doubt it is clear-
est when listened to in solitude. The ancestors say that God's
breath itself can be heard in quiet, and in stillness the Divine
whisper sounds as a trumpeting voice. This is what is meant by
the "thunder of silence." Many of these teachings eluded me,
but after much time hiking in the spectacular terrain of *Tshisimane*, I began to have an inkling of what the ancestors were
saying. The subtle aromas, colors, sunsets and sounds meditated me as I walked, and I needed no other formal spiritual
practice.

the source

The soul's language is learned by listening with the heart. It has many sounds including that of silence. Its eloquence is universal.

I already knew that incense burning could repel negative forces and invite the ancestors, and that many traditions used aroma to enhance access to the spirit world. As the Native Americans use sage, others cedar, so too do the *sangomas* burn impepho (Helichrysum) to thank and call the spirits.

There are many paths to the mystery wisdom exuding from the growing beings that surround us, from the color of the sky and from all still beings. It is impossible for the world to exist without fragrance, for our souls to survive without aroma. One must breathe deeply into the spirit flow. Only through the spirit self can we access the mystery which is itself spirit. The soul's sense must be fed.

These words affirmed why burning of incense would always remain part of my daily ritual to the ancestors, and that there is no better place to feed the soul's senses than pristine wilderness. This also was the teaching of the ancient Hebrew shamans, as well as the druids.

XI

Muti

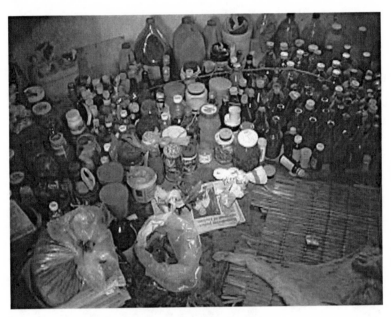

Sangoma's Muti bottles

DURING ALL THIS TIME I WAS FACED WITH THE EQUALLY huge task of learning the plants in this incredibly biodiverse area of the world. The Soutpansberg ecosystem boasts more than 600 trees and is as rich in flora as the much larger Kruger National Park. At first the task was daunting because all the trees looked the same to me. The botany I had studied during my first year of medicine in Johannesburg was a very distant and hazy memory. I set out to get various tree experts to come and walk

with me in the bush to identify the trees so I could have tree tags
made. We laid out many walks in the different ecosystems that
were edified by these tags. George and the botanist and I would
walk in the bush, identify and label the trees with the appropriate
standard tree numbers so that later we could affix aluminum tags
to them, including the Venda names. At first the specifics of their
identification seemed to elude me, but it was not long before I
could identify most of the medicinal trees in the area that we had
marked. To identify all of the trees would have been too great an
undertaking, so I decided to stick with those that had medicinal
or magical value. In the evenings and in my time off from building during the day, I would be at my computer summarizing all
the books that had been written on the medicinal properties of the
plants that were applicable to the area. I collated the information
together into an intelligible whole. This, together with the building and the hiking in the bush, kept me busy.

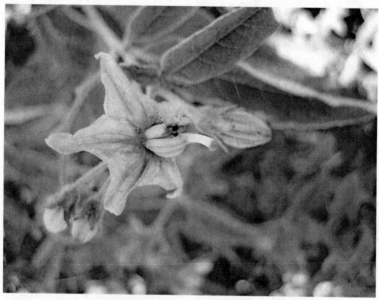

Solanum incanum or Poison apple
(Tandpynbos in Afrikaans, or toothache bush)

We were especially fortunate in having several different eco-systems at *Tshisimane*, giving us access to a plethora of medicinal plants. The land spanned montane, riverine and bushveld regions, with their differing vegetations. Some of the plants, such as the proteas in the montane areas, usually are found only in the more southern, cooler parts of South Africa. After a period of time we had a variety of different hikes plotted out so that folks could walk in the bush, view the labeled trees, and with the database learn their medicinal uses.

A great source of information for me was Dries Bester, a tour guide, environmental impact assessor and local tree expert, who had a special interest in their medicinal properties. He spoke several Bantu languages and knew many of the local *sangomas*. He helped me not only with the identifications, but also with the most important uses of the plants. Our research was later to materialize into a book on the medicinal trees and plants of the Soutpansberg. This later matured into another book, Healing Trees and Plants of the Lowveld, after we extended the data to include the southern part of the Kruger National Park. The Kruger Lowveld was more trafficked than the Soutpansberg and this book was more likely to be of interest because of the numerous bush lodges and the numbers of tourists who frequented the area. Dries was well acquainted with the Kruger flora as well as that of the Soutpansberg area. We enlisted the help of Rael Loon, who had access to pristine places in that region where we could complete the study. Rael is involved in ecotourism and, being especially interested in "People and Parks" as they relate to Tsonga culture in the Lowveld, he had a keen interest in medicinal plants.

I renewed my knowledge with Rael from time to time by walking in the Lowveld with local Tsonga guides who are

friends of his and who work for lodges in the region. The Soutpansberg contains most of the trees and plants that we had
covered in the previous book. With the help of Dries, it did not
take too much effort to fill in those medicinal Lowveld trees
that did not exist in the Soutpansberg. Overall the entire plant
project took several years of research and afforded the groups
who came to *Tshisimane* an extra dimension in understanding
the way medicinal plants work.

African lore teaches that there is a remedy for every eventuality, and although trees and plants are used for medical problems, they are also used for psycho-socio-spiritual problems as
well. There are medicines for luck, love, dreams, protection,
calling the ancestors and to prevent witchcraft, among others. I
realized that learning the plants was probably the main reason
the ancestors had sent me to the Soutpansberg. My knowledge
of plant medicines had been deficient during my initiation and
I was to rectify it at *Tshisimane.*

Part of Inward Bound's mission statement now was to research the medicinal values of the different plants. I learned
much about plant identification from botanists and books;
other ideas of how they worked were picked up slowly from
various *sangomas* during my stay. Traditional healers tend to
be secretive about their remedies, which often have been revealed to them by their own ancestors and hence are regarded
as "private." The game rangers and trackers in the Lowveld
were much more forthcoming in sharing information, as were
other non-*sangoma* folks who knew a lot from their parents and
grandparents, many of whom had been traditional healers.

Medicinal plants are the main source of medication for 80
percent of Southern Africa's black population. Pharmacological
evidence for their efficacy seemed scant due to limited research,

but there was no doubt that the medications worked. After my years of practical research at *Tshisimane*, I discovered that many of the plants had dozens of uses, sometimes conflicting. A certain plant might be used by one *sangoma* for constipation and by another for diarrhea. A tree used to cause abortion by one healer could be used to prevent it by another. I paid special attention to plants of power where there was pan-African use, even though they were used for differing complaints in various regions of the subcontinent.

The traditional healer is a master at enhancing the placebo effect. Placebo is the power of belief to heal, help or cure; nocebo is the power of belief to hurt, harm or even kill. In medicine it is well known that when a dummy medicine is given there is a positive effect at least 30% of the time. Medical research seeks to extract this effect to determine the actual power of the drug. Hence double blind studies are performed in which the patients are divided into two comparable groups, one getting the placebo and the other the real medicine. The groups and the researchers are "blinded" (hence doubly) by not knowing who received what, and so that the power of belief can be discounted. The pharmaceutical company would be looking for a beneficial effect well in excess of placebo's 30%.

It is possible that *sangomas*, with their ancestor-enhanced power, may be able to increase placebo well beyond 30% because they encourage their patients' trust in the rituals, the medicines and the ancestors. Rather than discounting placebo, they enhance it with their magic, whether it is uncannily accurate divinations, spectacular dancing, or even sometimes the ability to handle fire while in trance without getting burnt. The competence of the healer may have a lot to do with his or her skill in manipulating placebo, though a significant pharmacological action cannot be discounted.

One also has to take into account the power of the ancestral spirits invoked with a plant medicine or when a particular ritual is prescribed. The diagnosis is made from the spirit world either in trance, from a dream, or with the help of the divining bones, and the medicine dispensed may be in essence a password to the ancestors to effect a specific healing. The plant usage is often prescribed according to the "Law of Similars or Signatures." For instance, Kiaat, which has red bark, is used for menstrual and blood disorders. In this way, possibly, it is easier for the ancestral spirits to connect with the "password" of the *muti* to effect that particular healing. Animal products are also used for healing, but I did not study these. They also are usually prescribed according to the Law of Similars or Signatures, for instance, part of an elephant to give strength.

The Ancestors had stressed to us that all rituals and healing require a "container" which contains and magnifies the effect of the "blessing" transmitted by universal healing energy, which is really Divine love. In essence the container acts as a medium for the healing intentions of the *sangoma* for a particular therapeutic outcome that will be provided by the ancestors. It is analogous to the way that the bones provide a scaffold for the diagnostic insight coming from the spirit world. It is easier for spirit to work through some medium than without it. Every time a client uses the *muti* they are also giving their permission for a therapeutic intervention. Since free will is so important in the spirit world, "informed consent," as we would call it in medical jargon, is critical each time help is requested.

There are no trained healers who use all the plants in their area, and a practitioner becomes familiar with a set repertoire of plants found to be effective, or learned from a mentor, or from the ancestors. Many healers "dream" the plant that the patient will need. Healing, healer, patient, and "Spirit," or the ancestors, are inseparable in this indigenous healing wisdom. The whole is more than the sum of its parts. Extracting and concentrating components as is done in Western medicine, although often leading to powerful actions, also sometimes creates serious side effects.

One of the best examples of this can be seen in South America with extraction of cocaine from the coca leaf. When used holistically, the leaf has many beneficial alkaloids that work together not only to prevent and help high altitude sickness, but also to give energy and suppress the appetite. Its ubiquitous indigenous use in South America is helpful, as opposed to the abuse of the highly concentrated cocaine extract which has become so common in the West.

Safe dosages of these plants can only be decided by an experienced traditional healer, who not only knows where and when to collect the medicine, but also how to prepare it. Some plants used are highly toxic and the gap between therapeutic effectiveness and severe side effects, even death, is often very narrow.

It was for this reason, as well as the fact that as an M.D. I have many fine modern options available, that I was reluctant to use the plants systemically. I use them primarily topically and in baths for psycho-socio-spiritual maladies or "dis"-ease. Sometimes they are burnt or even smoked. However, I rely on my allopathic skills for most organic diseases unless Western medicine has failed to help the patient. Traditional healers would argue that all "dis"-ease will eventually lead to disease and that they go to the root of the problem rather than treating only its manifestations as we do in the West, and I would not argue with this.

In the past, collection of traditional medicines did not up-set the natural environment. Now *muti* traders tend to har-vest irresponsibly in order to satisfy a growing industry. These traders are only interested in profiteering and do not collect according to the time-honored ethics and principles of tradi-tional healers. For instance, if the plant or tree is killed, the medicine will not work and could even harm the harvester; medicine should not be collected from a plant previously used by another healer; roots must not be left exposed; trees should never be ring-barked; only enough for immediate use should be taken. The season, rainfall, and even the phase of the moon and so on, all need to be taken into account.

The Soutpansberg, being in the tropics, is rich in medici-nal plants whose healing potential has barely been tapped by Western science. I also learned that there is a huge difference between developing a relationship with a plant, harvesting it mindfully and then using it, as opposed to simply buying medicine from a *muti* market supported by the traders men-tioned above. Connecting with the ancestors, intention and integrity with plant usage is seminal, and offerings or a prayer are best made to the plant before harvesting. Many ancestors would prefer if possible that "their" medicines be consciously harvested, and if possible prepared by the *sangoma* or someone trusted by him or her. No mechanical devices can be used; ev-erything must be done by hand. I used to wonder why *muti* was so expensive and could even cost more than a divination until I learned how labor intensive the preparation can be. This is all the more so because roots and bark are usually used. These have to be cut up, dried, pounded and ground by hand and then sifted into a fine powder. In the Soutpansberg the most powerful *muti*s are also often in the most inaccessible places, and encounters with snakes and other hazards are part of the collector's job description.

My experience in California and Peru was that shamans and curanderos often would relate to the "spirit" in the plant. This did not seem to be part of the *sangoma* dialogue that I experienced, though it was clear they differentiated between plants that were "strong" and those that were not. Sometimes the most inauspicious and humble of plants were said to be "strong." The differing actions mentioned above probably have to do with the *sangoma's* relationship with his or her ancestral spirits and how they were directed, in and out of dreams, to use them. I found that this was also true for myself, and I would dream plants that I was instructed to use for a particular problem that I had not come across in my research. It seems clear that the spirit guides have a huge say in what a *sangoma* uses and have their own idiosyncratic ideas and preferences.

Of further interest to me, having spent several years with curanderos in Peru, was the absence of safe mind-altering plants in South Africa. Although I had benefited tremendously from imbibing some of these substances during my spiritual adventures in Peru, I never wanted to use any as part of my healing repertoire. San Pedro cactus had not done much for me, but the few times I had taken Ayahuasca in the Amazon had been life-changing. The vision I had of a house without a roof in the bushveld, that later proved to be *Tshisimane*, occurred during a ceremony with this "vision vine of the jungle." I gravitated away from Peruvian healers back to my roots in South Africa because I preferred the idea of using drumming, chanting and dancing to induce altered states of consciousness rather than entheogens. *Sangomas* mostly access the trance state purely with the use of drumming, dancing and chanting.

Datura is ubiquitous in the Lowveld but is not indigenous to South Africa. It is highly toxic and frequently lethal. The seeds, which contain high concentrations of hyoscine and atropine, are called "*malpitte*" in Afrikaans "seeds that make you mad"—and frequently cause death.

Certain Amaryllis species are also highly psychoactive and very dangerous, and have been used only by the older, more expert *sangomas* as the so-called "bioscope *muti*" ("bioscope" being an old South African term for a movie theater). I have heard stories of its effectiveness and toxicity but could never find a *sangoma* who knew how to use it or wanted to because it was so dangerous. The ritual comprises drinking a brew and then looking into a mirror. A vision of the solution to the problem you are searching for plays out like a movie in the mirror due to the profound mind-altering effect of the plant.

After I became familiar with the Soutpansberg flora I began to focus on the magical and medicinal plants of California. When I would return to Santa Barbara I extended the same principles I had learned in South Africa to my home environment. I focused at first on learning the plants of power in California's Central Coast, an amazingly bio-diverse region. Being mainly plants and bushes, these medicines are much easier to harvest and process than the tree medicines that predominate in the Soutpansberg. On occasion I would also dream California plants. Now I could fully function as a *sangoma* not only in South Africa but also in California.

XII

Bad Neighbors

SOON AFTER I BEGAN THE BUILDING OF *TSHISIMANE*, I HAD
a powerful dream that appeared twice in one night. The
dream told me in no uncertain terms that I needed to buy the
adjacent farm, Calitzdorp, which had been for sale for some
time. I was not sure of the reason for this but thought that it
might be because of someone unsavory taking it over if I did
not. We already had an unpleasant character to contend with,
Hendrik, who owned the farm below Calitzdorp. I also had an
ominous dream at the time about lights from the village below
"spreading" up the mountain towards *Tshisimane*. The dream
about Calitzdorp was to prove auspicious.

I already had enough land in the purchase of Uniondale –
1500 acres. I really did not need another 1500 and did not have
the money for the purchase. However, around that time our
foundation was given a generous donation. Being convinced
about the ancestors' foresight I took out a second mortgage on
my home in Santa Barbara and bought the property.

Calitzdorp had been owned and developed in previous years
by the local dentist. He had also been the mayor of Makhado
and was now deceased. His son had inherited the farm. The son
had no real interest in the land and had emigrated to Canada,
leaving it under the management of Hendrik. The agreement
was that in return for looking after the farm, Hendrik could

harvest the macadamia nut trees. In fairness to Hendrik, this was now the domain of the baboon troop that foraged the trees and there were very few nuts to be had.

Hendrik was a colorful man. Two of his qualities were a distinct lack of integrity and a bad temper. He was a big burly man, overweight, and had worked for the local police station for many years. Now retired, he had retained his connection to his buddies in the force and allowed them to graze their cattle on his land and also hunt there on occasion. This gave him a lot of clout with that station. He was a tough character and had been using his position as manager of Calitzdorp to his own advantage.

Since retiring, he was farming cattle and a few assorted vegetables on his land. He hunted game on his own property and that he was entitled to do, but he had also been poaching game on Calitzdorp. This continued whenever I was away in California, even after I purchased the land. He had also been harvesting lumber (including protected trees) and selling the wood to improve his income. Richard, who now worked for me, had done part-time jobs for Hendrik and had been involved in the tree felling and selling. He told me he had hardly been paid and was essentially working for food.

Since my arrival we'd had an ongoing problem with Hendrik, who refused to restrain his dogs from attacking the workers who walked the road to get to the farms above Calitzdorp. In fact he encouraged them to harass the men. The macadamia nut farm and homestead at Calitzdorp were in total disrepair, the trees were uncared for, and the irrigation system was now useless. The baboons not only ate whatever little was left of the macadamia crop, but had also ravaged the once beautiful house and torn the thatch roofs apart. Hendrik had also cut down some exotic trees around the homestead, including part of a magnificent coral tree that had fallen on the roof of the house in the process, partially demolishing it. In short, when I acquired Calitzdorp it was a mess.

Lorne, a good friend of mine, was interested in the farm and brought his farmer uncle to look at it. His assessment was that it would take several hundred thousand rand to restore the macadamia plantation and even then, there was little hope of containing the baboons. Rupert's uncle Boet, a macadamia farmer from the eastern Soutpansberg, gave the same prognosis. He had known the dentist-mayor who had established the macadamias. Boet related how the local farmers had been amused at the dentist's attempts, especially because the trees he chose were of inferior quality. He had also refused to acknowledge that the rainfall on the western part of the mountain was inadequate to sustain a macadamia crop. I overheard Boet politely whispering to Rupert in Afrikaans, "Please tell your friend Dave not to try and farm these macadamias." I listened to this advice, but the baboons did not. In fact they fully agreed with the ancestors' wisdom below:

Do not be deterred by the bitter skin of sweet fruit nor discouraged by the hard shells of succulent nuts.

The baboons were undaunted, but for me a macadamia project would be too difficult a nut to crack. Macadamia shells are extremely hard, but the baboons had no trouble cracking them with their teeth and enjoying the proceeds. Furthermore, dogs did not seem to be a deterrent, and even a large dog is no match for a grown male baboon. The cunning of baboons is legendary, and the realtor who sold me the farm enlightened me further about the macadamia-baboon problem. He related how a farmer friend of his, in frustration, had erected an electrical fence. While patrolling it one day he came across a large male baboon who had lifted the wire to allow the rest of the troop to go in under it to feast. The baboon was unperturbed by the shocks he was receiving during his altruistic endeavor. Another farmer told me of a pet baboon near the Blouberg who had been taught to drive a tractor and about how another had even been trained to work on the railway line.

Baboons can be ingenious in their determination to find food wherever they can. Breaking and entering is not beyond them in their attempts to do this. A friend left her house in a game reserve tightly closed, the windows secured, and all the outside doors locked. They left the house safe and sound, or so they thought. When they returned much later, the house was in shambles. The baboons had scrutinized the property and found one window which, unnoticed by the owner, was minimally ajar. They maneuvered it until it was open, broke the fly screen and burst in. They ransacked the kitchen, scattering food at random, and then vandalized the rest of the house, trailing their spoils and leaving their "calling cards" behind wherever they went. Baboons can even manage to unzip tents and undo latches in their quest for illicit groceries.

A neighbor told me of how she had found a baboon in her tented lodge. She yelled at him in a successful effort to chase him out. As he left the tent he had unzipped to get in, he politely zipped it closed again! Fortunately this kind of baboon trickery only happened once at *Tshisimane.*

I was convinced the baboon battle was one I could not win now that I was the not-so-proud owner of primate-controlled Calitzdorp. We finally cut down all the macadamias and restored the land to its previous wild beauty – the best thing we could have done. The baboons, I imagined, had enough pleasure ravaging the mango trees down at Calitzdorp and the grove next to the *Tshisimane* house. During my seven years there I never got a chance to eat even one of these; I always had to buy them in the supermarkets of Makhado.

When we began to clean up the property we had a few surprises. We discovered that the dentist-mayor had been making moonshine (*mampoor* in Afrikaans) from the prickly pear cactus fruit he had planted all around. We found numerous old fridges hidden in the bush where he had stored the *mampoor* before selling it in Makhado. The more I learnt about him, the more intrigued I became with this colorful character. We even set up a little plaque on the antiquated macadamia nut shelling machine to honor his ancestral spirit. Calitzdorp must have been a compelling farm in its heyday, with magnificent views of the mountains to the north from the homestead. Abandoned farms like these are all too prevalent in the remote areas of South Africa, where hardy farmers set up a life for themselves and then for one or another reason, political or practical, were forced to leave the dream for which they had worked so hard.

By this time land claims had surfaced on *Tshisimane*, even though they had not existed when I purchased the farm. My attorney had checked with Land Claims in Polokwane before the purchase of Calitzdorp and I had been assured there were none and would be none. It became clear that many land claims were being insinuated after the cutoff date for a land claim to be lodged. It was also apparent that now that *Tshisimane* was in the process of being developed, there was a much greater motivation to claim the land. At the time I mistakenly thought that not being legal, the claim was frivolous, and I was not particularly worried about it.

After the purchase of Calitzdorp, I tried to ensure that Hendrik would no longer come and poach on the farm or harvest wood. This was made clear to him from the get-go. We had already had some exchanges with him that were extremely unpleasant. He refused to return a derelict trailer and sundry items that belonged to Calitzdorp until three of us came down the mountain to retrieve them with the tractor. He released them only after an ugly encounter and not until we paid him R250 for an axle that he said he had installed at his own expense. When we drove up the mountain with the trailer, Richard informed me that he was the one who had found and installed the axle, which had cost nothing. Richard also told me that Hendrik had been asking him for Calitzdorp's hand winch. It was a highly desirable item he had been searching for but, fortunately for us, could not find. Richard, who suspected this would happen, had hidden it in the bush. He located it and it proved invaluable to us during the building.

Henry would intermittently bring supplies for the tractor. Due to the horrendous road, he would off-load diesel and the rest at the bottom of the mountain for us to pick up later with the tractor and trailer. On one occasion, a 44-gallon drum of diesel was found to be half empty when we picked it up. One of Hendrik's workers admitted seeing him siphoning the drum. Hendrik had been reported to the police by neighbors on more than one occasion for cutting down endangered trees. However, because of his police connections, except for a warning, nothing much ever came of it.

There was a Lister diesel generator belonging to Calitzdorp which Hendrik had removed and installed on his farm before I took ownership. When it broke down he sent it in for repair to Makhado. He refused to pay the 7000 rand for the repairs and the engine was impounded at the engineer's workshop. Although now that I had solar I had no use for a generator, I decided to pay the 7000 rand and bring it back to Calitzdorp as a back-up system in case we developed the new farm. This was not an easy task because of the weight. The Lister is a real workhorse and has the reputation of lasting forever. After loading the engine onto the back of my pickup with the shop's winch, we drove off to the Calitzdorp homestead and up the neglected road that was now little more than a track, to deposit it. Only three of us knew about this – George, Richard and myself. We used the tractor to get the diesel off the pickup and then the three of us were barely able to scoot the heavy engine along the concrete floor into the house. We covered it with the canopy of my pickup so that it could not be seen. We locked the house and I assumed the engine would be safe. I left for California, and on my return when I went to check on it, it was gone. We suspected it was Hendrik who had stolen the diesel, although we had no proof.

At that time Richard had left my employment because he, like Dennis, had also begun to drink heavily. George suspected that he had informed Hendrik of the Lister and together they may have planned the heist. Hendrik had lent Richard money to buy his house and possibly this was a way of appeasing him for the unpaid loan, since Hendrik was threatening to repossess Richard's home. George told me that Hendrik had a second farm and imagined he had taken the Lister to use at that location. On the other hand Hendrik may have had nothing to do with the theft, but it had clearly been an inside job.

I lodged a police report at the local station to have it on record in spite of the fact that I knew it was futile. We never found out where the Lister ended up or who had stolen it, in spite of police assurances that they would track down the offender. For security reasons we installed a relative of George's in the Calitzdorp house and allowed him to graze his cattle there. I rarely used the property except for hiking or harvesting *muti*. Calitzdorp had a spectacular riverine section with natural springs and an interesting cave. It was a good day's walk to hike along the southern crest of Tshismane and drop down into this area and then hike back to the homestead. Every now and again, with suitable groups, we would enjoy the challenging trek. Most of the Calitzdorp terrain was more open and flat, and did not have the spiritual power that was *Tshisimane's*.

George would get periodic reports from his relative on Calitzdorp about Hendrik cruising around in his *bakkie* on my land, especially when I was in California. In addition to allowing the local police to graze their cattle on his land, we suspected that Hendrik invited them to come and poach at Calitzdorp from time to time. Most of the game on Hendrik's farm had been shot out. George reported hearing an occasional shot coming from below while I was away.

On one occasion I was driving back from Makhado past Hendrik's farm on the dirt road close to the Sand River when I saw two police *bakkies* parked on the side. Just as I was about to pass them by, I saw one of the officers come out of the bush trying his best to conceal a semi-automatic weapon. I could see the barrel of it sticking out before he got into the driver's seat. I drove by with a friendly wave, pretending I had seen nothing. I felt intuitively that the party was heading to Calitzdorp to scout out what game they could find. Calitzdorp was at least twenty minutes' drive down the mountain from the *Tshisimane* homestead, and by the time one could have responded to the sound of a shot – these folks were expert marksmen – any poacher would be long gone with his trophy.

I decided to stop and wait once I entered the Calitzdorp gate and fence line. I hid my *bakkie* in the bush and watched the road. After about 45 minutes it was getting close to sunset and I thought that if they were to arrive, staying any longer might not be such a good idea. I drove back up to the homestead and told George what I had seen. Early the next morning we both drove down to the Calitzdorp house, where George's cousin confirmed that two police vehicles had entered at dusk, driven around, probably looking for bushbuck, and then had left. We established this by identifying the vehicles' tracks, which were the same as those I had seen when I passed them by that day at the Sand River. There was not much more I could do about this other than to try to catch them red-handed, which also would probably have been dangerous.

The previous owner of Dundee, Robert, whose farm I had nearly bought, had retained a small piece of land around the homestead that he would visit from time to time. The rest of Dundee had been sold off to the new neighbors, who could not have been a nicer replacement. My experiences with Robert in the past were alluded to early on in the story, when I first approached him about buying Dundee and had found him to be untrustworthy. I continued to be bothered by him after I bought Uniondale and Calitzdorp. There were two access roads to his homestead, the one he had always used that bypassed my lands, and the other that was the longer way around through Lesheba. Due to the poaching problem, we had decided to lock the entrance gate to Calitzdorp, and everyone who used the easement to the top of the mountain had a key to the gate except Robert, who had been disagreeable and difficult to contact. We had left numerous messages and George had spoken to him about giving him a key, but to no avail. Robert, instead, chose to take a grinder with him in his *bakkie*, and every time he came to the gate he would either cut the lock off or sever the chain. Eventually, out of frustration, together with Rupert, I went to see him in his Polokwane office. I addressed the concern to his secretary. I could see him listening to me through a partially open office door, but he made no attempt to come out. I gave his secretary the key to the new lock and she said she would pass it on. Robert continued to cut the chain and we gave up trying to lock the gate.

XIII

projects and plans

You will give importance to the unnecessary until you
come to realize it is wasteful of your time and of yourself.
Then you will dare to stop and do only what is needful to
be more of what is truly you.

W HEN I FIRST PURCHASED *TSHISIMANE* I HAD MANY IDEAS.
The mission statement of the Inward Bound Healing
Journeys foundation was to build a center in Southern Africa
to validate and research indigenous healing knowledge, especially the use of medicinal plants. I planned to bring in different
sangomas and healers to establish a model to document the practices of the local peoples. This included the Venda, the Tsonga
and the local Pedi, a Sotho group who were close by. In this way
the local tribes could have their healing traditions, which had
been mainly orally transmitted, validated and documented. A
museum to honor this wisdom had been part of the plan.

The idea of a *sangoma* think tank was to prove a dismal
failure, since I was somewhat naïve in my understanding of
the way *sangomas* work. I come from a medical background
in which information is always shared freely. I thought that
this would also be the case with traditional healers but soon
learned that there was a significant amount of secrecy among
my *sangoma* "colleagues." *Sangomas* are reluctant to share their

wisdom with other *sangomas* for several reasons. One is related, no doubt, to jealousy and competitiveness. The other is the fear of being bewitched by their own medicines or techniques, or that their practices could be neutralized or even turned against them by those who had evil inclinations. This unspoken principle was something I failed to understand in the early days, resulting in considerable disappointment in my quest. There were other issues as well.

On one occasion I met up with a *sangoma* from the Blouberg, a magnificent mountain range west of the Soutpansberg. This *sangoma* lived at the foot of the mountain and stated that he used the Blouberg to get his medicinal plants. I went to his small village, picked him up and brought him to *Tshisimane* to walk with him in the bush. After several hours he identified one or two plants that he said he knew. When I asked him about the medicinal plants of power we encountered along our walk, such as a pepper bark tree, he would say, "No, these trees, they do not occur on the Blouberg, I do not know them. You must come to the Blouberg and I will show you the medicines that I use, the trees that I use that only grow there. Your trees are different."

A year later I took him up on his offer. A group of us went with him up the Blouberg, spent an evening on the top, and then trekked back down. Blouberg is a majestic range with a daunting profile and is rich in medicinal plants. It was clear from the outset that all the plants and trees, including all the plants of power that were at *Tshisimane*, were also in the Blouberg. The Blouberg *sangoma* rushed ahead on the trail and seemed unavailable for questions. At first I thought that he was just reluctant to give me any information about the plants he used. En route, however, when we stopped at a pepper bark tree, he was unable to identify it. I realized then that his behavior rather reflected his lack of knowledge about the plants and his embarrassment, though I cannot discount an element of secrecy as well. I assumed he was probably buying his medicines from other *sangomas* or traders, which, having already been harvested, would be non-distinct. If he purchased the bulbs, roots or bark he would not necessarily know how to identify them in the field. When I eventually gave him a ride home to his village, he tried to redeem himself from being "missing in action" on the hike. He took me into his house and showed me various powdered medicines that he used, but I suspect these were bought rather than self-gathered.

This was my first experience with the so-called "think tank" idea of inviting *sangomas* to *Tshisimane* to share their knowledge. George confirmed my suspicions later, after he had gone through his own *sangoma* initiation. He told me that the *sangoma* who was his mentor, and others that lived in the village, knew very little about the trees. My suspicion since then is that even those who harvest and prepare their own *muti* probably work only with a small repertoire of plants that they may or may not mix for differing effects.

I have a good friend, Mpata, who is an advocate for preserving the fast-disappearing Venda traditions. She had built a Venda cultural center to support and validate Venda ethnicity. She was also dedicated to preserving sacred Venda sites that were being developed and decimated. I often used her expertise to enlighten my groups. Her father had been a *sangoma* and the family was renowned in Venda, having close family links to the famous chief, Makhado, who fought and defeated the Boers. She was a direct descendant of Chief Makhado, and of royal blood. Mpata is a lovely woman of great integrity and proud of her lineage. She always dresses beautifully in Venda traditional clothing to support her heritage. She is a tour guide and has interesting stories to tell about her people.

Makhado was called "the Lion of the North" by the Afrikaners. Makhado had defeated them and their Swazi allies, as well as the Boers (Afrikaners), who were forced to leave Venda for awhile. This humiliating defeat haunted President Kruger and was unprecedented in the Boer history of victories against the various African tribes on their great trek northwards. The Afrikaners eventually returned and re-populated Venda after poisoning Makhado and finally defeating the Venda. The local town of Louis Trichardt was recently renamed Makhado, in honor of the great chief.

Mpata and I worked together video-documenting the stories of the elders, recording traditional Venda recipes, and filming what was left of their sacred places. Knowing my interest in *muti* she brought an herbalist, Peter, along with her uncle, to spend a weekend at *Tshisimane*. George and I, Mpata and Peter walked around *Tshisimane* for two full days, identifying different plants and attempting to talk about their medicinal values. George, who knew many of the medicinal trees from his grandfather, walked with us in the bush. For the first few hours, the herbalist walked around instructing us on the uses of several of the medicinal trees. He was clearly knowledgeable. However, after an hour or two, he became quite silent. When we would walk in an area full of other medical trees, I would ask him, "What about these trees? Do they have any medicinal action?" He would reply, "No, there is no medicine here." This continued throughout the morning. Puzzled, I took George aside and asked him what was going on. He said in Afrikaans, "Hy hou" – he is holding back, he is concealing, he is not telling you what he knows.

Mpata, herself, knew a lot of the plants and pointed out a wild yam plant that was well known in Venda to be toxic and dangerous. The crushed bulb causes a zombie-like state if ingested. It inhibits motor function and, in large doses, causes paralysis. Food liberally laced with the tuber had been used to bait, immobilize and catch baboons due to this unique action. Mpata related how the Venda had used it when anticipating a Swazi attack. The Venda warriors had cooked up cauldrons of corn meal (mielie pap) and laced them liberally with the dried powder from the tuber of these plants. They pretended to have been taken by surprise on the arrival of the Swazi warriors, and ran away. The Swazis, seeing the hot food, decided to sit down and take advantage of the meal. Later when they lay there temporarily paralyzed from the effects of the plant, though still awake, the Venda warriors came back and dispatched them.

On another occasion I invited a group of white *sangomas* to come and visit, and was met with the same frustrations. I would share the knowledge that I had learned over the years from my research, but it was not met with much reciprocity. When I would ask them about particular plants and what they used them for, they would avoid the question or tell me quite frankly, "This is a secret that our teacher does not allow us to disclose." During their visit I developed an upper respiratory tract infection. One of them volunteered to give me a concoction of six different plants that she had brought and assured me it would fix me in no time. She would not disclose the ingredients. Unwisely, I agreed to take it, and ended up with a terrible migraine for the next twelve hours. It was at this stage that my attempts for a medicinal plant think tank came to an end.

Although George trusted me and we developed a close bond and friendship, it was clear that in the beginning he, also, was not disclosing all the information that he knew. Maybe this was his way of not giving away all of his knowledge and personal power. There was one particular plant renowned in Venda for bringing good luck. Every time I would come to *Tshisimane* I would ask George when he was going to take me to find the plant. On each occasion he would say, "No, no, it is very far." When I would ask how far, how many hours' walk, he would say, "Oh, it would be all day and be difficult to come back the same day." Eventually, after a year or two of this conversation, I insisted on going regardless of the time and distance. He said, "Come and I will show you." Within 100 yards of the house he pointed out a small shrub to me and said, "That is the plant." It had been there all the time, but he had been reluctant to share the information.

Andries, who lived nearly two hours' drive away, was always available for consultation. He had a wealth of experience and knowledge, especially when it came to countering witchcraft and using *muti*. I would bring Andries to *Tshisimane* to dig for *muti* and he always seemed to be forthcoming with his recipes. He would walk in the bush with his wives and they would dig out roots from various plants and tell us what they were used for. However, I learned in time that there were other plants that I did not know about that were being added to these main ingredients, that he did not disclose. When I was back in California, George would drive quite frequently back and forth to visit Andries for help, and as trust grew, Andries would gradually impart some of this secret knowledge to him, and then George would share it with me on my return. By then we both realized that more than likely, for safety's sake, there would probably always be at least one plant that Andries added that we would not know about.

In addition to the *sangoma* think tank there were many other ideas. One was to reach out to the local village at the bottom of the mountain and provide its clinic with medical supplies. Direct Relief International (DRI) had generously sponsored the small clinic we had at *Tshisimane*, and was prepared to help in the surrounding area as well. This idea also proved to be a failure. DRI promised that as long as it could get an import tax exemption it was happy to supply not only the local clinic, but also the tertiary care hospital in nearby Elim. My attempts were met with frustration, both at the clinical level and even at the administrative level at both places. I would leave forms for the officials to fill out for the medical supplies and equipment they needed, only to come back later to find they had not been completed. I would complete the forms on their behalf, but they would not be submitted or cleared at a higher level. The tax exemptions requested also were not forthcoming.

Elim was a compelling teaching hospital that reminded me of the days I had studied medicine and specialized in surgery in Johannesburg in the 1960s and '70s. Nevertheless, it was short on medicines, supplies and equipment. I could not get things moving there either, however, in spite of generous promises of X-ray equipment, surgical instruments and drugs from DRI. Even taking the offer to the head of surgery at Elim was ineffective. At one stage, one of the CEOs of the hospital, a woman, was particularly motivated to make things happen, but unfortunately she became ill. She was replaced, and the project dissipated. She had been keen for me to sign on part-time as a urology consultant since they had no urologist on the faculty, but when she left I decided against it.

In the meantime I had also formulated some other ideas for *Tshisimane*, none of which materialized. The ancestors seemed only interested in the indigenous healing aspects and no other doors opened for me.

Another failed idea was to develop an outdoor leadership school for the local kids in the villages below. I invited a friend, Mungai, from Kenya, to help with the project. Some years previously Mungai had been my instructor at the National Outdoor Leadership School (NOLS), the largest outdoor school in the world, which at that time was also operating in Kenya. I had spent four weeks trekking around Mount Kenya and the Masai Mara area with him and was very impressed with his abilities. He is a wilderness expert skilled in every aspect of outdoor technology.

We decided we would spend three weeks working out a trans-Soutpansberg trail for our part of the mountain range. We devised a trail from one farm to the next, where youngsters from the local schools, birding enthusiasts and other hikers could spend up to five days crossing a section of this stunning wilderness. Ian Gaiger from Lajuma, west of *Tshisimane*, was very supportive of the idea, as were most of the other farmers in that area. One of the farmers objected on the grounds that it would increase poaching if youth from the village gained access to his lands. This required that we divert the trail through more difficult and less scenic terrain. Nevertheless, with the help of the other farmers in the area we did lay out a trail on paper with places to sleep along the way. However, that was as far as we got, for reasons related to land claims, which were to occupy my attentions shortly after the idea was conceived. Even when I visit there today, the local farmers remain disappointed that it did not materialize. Nevertheless, we had a great time researching the trail and discovering places I would never otherwise have seen.

I turned my attentions to another idea not long after I said farewell to Mungai. I applied for grants for a cultural village that would be housed on the lower farm at Calitzdorp. This would have afforded employment for the villagers below, but no grants materialized.

My main hope had been that I would be able to get interest and help in doing research on some of the powerful medicinal plants that were not easily found in the rest of the country and were not well known. Many of the major medicinal plants in South Africa had already been studied. However, one of my neighbors, who had far more financial resources than I did, liked my idea and decided to run with it while I was in California. When I came back I learned that he now had an ethnobotanist living on site and that he already had a research project underway. Since I was there only part of the year, I decided to let this plan go as well.

Abundance is not an achievement of the acquisitive, but rather a legacy of the perceptive, a realization of plenty — not an acquiring of more.

I already had my hands full with feeling my own way and developing my personal relationship with the plants. With time it became clear to me that these "dead ends" had never been the real reason I needed to be in the Soutpansberg. When I would return to California, the dream work with Maryellen continued. The information coming sometimes almost every night to the two of us from the ancestors kept me on track with my true mission and destiny path, in spite of my curious nature and tendency to wander away from my purpose.

Hence what transpired from 2002 to 2009 was a deepening of my knowledge of *sangoma* medicine, and especially of medicinal plants. I was fortunate in having George on hand to help me. His knowledge of the trees had grown, and as he started to learn the English names, I slowly picked up the Venda equivalents. Furthermore George enabled me to access more deeply the mindset of this rich culture. Much of the time we were the only two people at *Tshisimane* and I would often spend my leisure time chatting with him about Venda ways of thinking and their customs.

I noted from these experiences that when the work I was doing was in line with my true mission, all gates seemed to open for me. However, when it was not, the ancestors chose not to assist and support. It was as though when Maryellen and I would review the dream sayings again and again in California, I could hear them explaining to me why it was that I had so many frustrations and roads that led to disappointment. The sayings, even if sometimes in retrospect, reassured me that in fact I had not "failed." I recognized with time that ...

God does not measure results, only the purity of one's intent and the fervor of one's effort.

and also ...

Whatever does not help you be more of you, lures you to be less of you!

and to ...

Be patient with yourself, kind to yourself and, above all, release yourself from what you are not accountable. You must be free to be yourself. Do not be captive to the demands of false duty.

The ancestors indulged my dream to have a place in the bush, but it became clear they were not interested in a cultural village, indigenous museums, a wilderness school or a *sangoma* think tank. They were, however, interested in my deepening my knowledge of healing and its opposite, witchcraft, and delving into plant medicines for healing rather than for pharmaceutical research. If there was even a hint that my activities were a distraction or pandering to my ego, a lack of their support was assured. When the ancestors were displeased with my direction, the power of free will disallowed them to actually hamper my progress, but neither were they obligated to help. Theirs were not acts of commission to deter, but rather omission to assist, which accounted for my coming up against the barriers they may otherwise have been able to remove. I could imagine I heard them chiding me.

> *As fame can enslave, so can the costs of money*
> *impoverish. Make sure the need is worth the price.*
> *To overpay can rob the self.*

Although money and prestige had never been my motivation, there may have been an element of "fame-seeking," in the broadest sense of the word, which was captivating me. However, there should never have been any concern on my behalf to have made *Tshisimane* anything other than what it became. Although Mabata had thought that the project could have been of considerable interest to the government, which was interested in an African renaissance, this was not to be. The only thing that did materialize that somewhat pandered to my ego was a visit by the South African Broadcasting Corporation as I was about to close *Tshisimane* down. They wanted to do an hour-long TV segment on my story. This, for unknown reasons, was given the title of "Wounded Healer" and can be viewed on my website. They even came to Santa Barbara to film the white *sangoma*-surgeon who worked in two different worlds.

> *Bestow blessings, refuse burdens. What makes you beholden enslaves you. What makes you grateful blesses you. What you touch touches you. What you let touch you, enhances or diminishes.*

XIV

Employees, friends and guests

EXCEPT FOR GEORGE THERE WAS AN ONGOING PROBLEM with staff. It always seemed to start off well. George respected my *sangoma* status, understood the spiritual nature of our project and realized we were there to do work for the ancestors. As time went on, George became more and more preoccupied with dreams. It seemed that in these dreams he was being called to become a *sangoma* by his deceased *sangoma* grandfather.

As a youth, George had gone through the standard male initiation that most Venda youth were required to endure. This was a significant event, because it had been at a time when initiations were done in the "old way" by the elders. Since circumcision was always a vital part of the initiation it was important to know the medicines and the rituals to use to protect against witchcraft, bleeding, infection and other maladies, including death. Unfortunately, death and serious complications have become quite common today because of circumcisions done by inexpert *sangomas*, charlatans or persons who have none of the old knowledge, so much so that many parents now prefer to go to a medical doctor just for the procedure. Since the nature of the initiation was secret, I never really got to hear all the details from George, but this is what I learned over my years in Venda.

Youngsters would be taken into the bush for up to a three-month period in the winter. Their only possessions were a blanket and a food bowl. Their food consisted of corn meal porridge (mielie pap), supplemented at times with food only from the bush. Temporary huts were constructed and there was a pole in the center of the encampment that represented "Grandfather." The initiates would dance and kneel submissively around the pole. A ceremonial fire was maintained at all times. At the conclusion of the schooling, the boys were circumcised. Originally this was performed by a Lemba expert using a sharp reed. (For more details on the Lemba tribe, refer to the Appendix.) Later a blade was substituted and Venda *sangomas*, such as George's father, officiated entirely. After the procedure the boys would have to stand in cold water in the river to staunch the bleeding. Later special medicinal plants would be applied to prevent infection. At the closure of the initiation process the youth had to go to the river and "wash their childhood away." They then covered themselves with red ochre so they could not be easily recognized on their return home. They returned home as men, singing their initiation songs. On the occasions when one would perish, the boy would be buried next to one of the shelters and the site covered with rocks. Only his food bowl would be returned to his parents.

The fact that George had been initiated showed in his toughness and stamina, his aptitude in the bush, his ability to read animal tracks and to understand what was going on in the ecosystem. It also showed in his general attitude towards life. I was less fortunate with some of the other workers, who had bypassed this ancient tradition. The initiation process is still highly regarded in Venda today, and those who have not been initiated cannot participate in tribal court or marital hearings.

When I would return to *Tshisimane* and notice a lot of trash lying about I would try to instill a wilderness and ancestor consciousness in the employees by saying, "If President Mandela were coming to visit, would you not want this place to be nice and clean?" They would answer in the affirmative and then I would add, "The ancestors are even bigger than Mandela, so you should do the same for them. This is their place." This had the effect I wanted and the aesthetic nature of *Tshisimane* became much easier to maintain.

The first employee, Dennis, was extremely enthusiastic at first, but it was not long before George informed me that, when I was away, he was drinking and would not show up for work. George was the foreman and when he would take Dennis to task for his behavior Dennis would become abusive, and would not listen in spite of drawing his pay. When I came back to *Tshisimane* I had to fire him.

There was another significant event involving Dennis soon after he began to drink. It occurred at the time when I still trusted him. One day after coming up the mountain with all the supplies from Makhado, I realized that my wallet had disappeared. I could not place exactly where I had lost it. I went back to the hardware store where I had bought all my supplies but no wallet had been found there. I retraced my steps to all the places I had been to during the day and could not find it anywhere. I asked George and I asked Dennis, who had helped me unpack the car, and both of them said they had not seen it. My credit cards had been in the wallet, and a considerable amount of cash. The biggest nuisance was the loss of my driver's license. This problem manifested later that trip and resulted in my inability to rent a car on my return to Los Angeles. I had to wait hours for a bus and then endure a two-hour bus ride back home after a grueling 30-hour flight.

I suspected that Dennis might have been the one who was responsible for its "loss" because I often left my wallet on the car seat while driving, but I had no proof of it. Much later, after he was fired, I found the wallet underneath some supplies packed away in the back of a closet. The credit cards and license were still there, but the money was gone.

George and I both noticed over the years that if anyone at *Tshisimane* "misbehaved," the karmic consequences of their actions seemed to come around quickly to meet them. Around the time Dennis began to "turn," a strange thing happened to him. He lived in a tiny two-roomed house with his wife and two children. One room served as a bedroom where he and his wife slept, and the other as a kitchen, eating and living area where the children slept. Fortunately, the weekend the event occurred, his wife and children had left for a visit to her mother. George told me this was because of an altercation, since Dennis was now drinking heavily on his weekends off.

That Monday, Dennis came to work with his forearm quite severely burned. Fortunately the burn was superficial, but it was extensive. He was puzzled and related how a fire had spontaneously broken out in the kitchen area while he was sleeping. The source of this spontaneous combustion appeared to be a few dirty rags that possibly had some kerosene on them. He assured us he had not been drinking and was dismayed by what happened. He was adamant that there were no candles or lanterns burning at the time he had gone to sleep. The kids would almost certainly have been burned if they had been home. Dennis had managed to put out the fire, but not before many of their belongings were incinerated. The house, made out of bricks with a corrugated iron roof, survived.

I was concerned that the burn might get infected and turn from a superficial to a deep one. I put antibacterial silvadene ointment on it and dressed it every day to protect it from the work environment. I noticed several days later that Dennis was digging a hole without his dressing on. When I asked him why, he said he did not think my medicine was any good so he had gone to see a *sangoma*, who had given him something to rub on it. This *sangoma* had told Dennis that he could do anything he wanted to do, with no coverings over the burn to get in his way. I asked what was in the medicine. He was vague and said that it had various plants mixed with python fat, but he did not know which plants. I was concerned, but said nothing. A week later the burn was almost completely healed and Dennis was going about his work uneventfully. I was humbled. Over the years many of my Western ideas were overturned, including this example. The *muti* he used defied my concepts on the dangers of soil bacteria, tetanus, secondary infection of burns, and my medical training with its sophisticated repertoire of medications.

By this time I had already taken on Richard, who was a hard worker and who filled the lapses in Dennis's work schedule. He, like Dennis, also seemed to be fine in the beginning, until he, too, began to drink with the proceeds of his salary and had to be fired. It was just before that happened that the Lister diesel engine mysteriously disappeared from Calitzdorp.

Richard was replaced with Simon, an affable sort of a fellow, not particularly smart, but incredibly strong and hardworking. At this stage I was quite cynical about employees, and when I would ask George about their future prognoses he would always say in Afrikaans, *"Nou is hy reg maar miskien hy sal draai"* – "At the moment he is okay, but maybe he will turn." This statement turned out to be wise counsel. George did not drink, and fully understood the impact of alcohol that frequently took somebody from being a gainful employee to being unmanageable. The same later proved true for Simon, who also "turned" and had to leave the employment. His father sometimes delivered him angrily to work after a weekend of bingeing as if he had been a naughty child. At first I thought the father was looking out for his son, until George told me that he was taking a sizable amount from Simon's wages for himself. Maybe Simon had decided to drink it all before his father got his hands on it.

I remember being advised by a black friend of mine about how to select an employee. He held a very important government administrative position, and this is what he suggested. He said I should line up the prospective applicants and ask them one question. "Those among you who do not drink, step forward!" In his experience, most of the group would step forward. He then told me that I should employ the ones who did not step forward and were honest enough to admit that they drank.

At this stage the buildings at *Tshisimane* were completed, and mostly only maintenance was required. George could handle this quite well on his own. The healing hut that had been partially open was now enclosed in canvas walls with netting for windows, secure from baboons and larger animals. The ritual bath was fully functional and the open lapa was perfect for doing yoga with groups. A separate area had been landscaped for *braais*. The roads had been improved, and paths around the homestead were delineated with the circles that had been made from the cut eucalyptus trees. We had also built a labyrinth, and a medicine wheel, to bring in different spiritual components to the healing center. The database for the plants was complete. Furnishings, though rustic, were comfortable, and cupboards were in place.

The kitchen had been upgraded to be able to cook for at least twelve people. The solar was working, the wind pump added to the energy when there was no sun, and all in all the design proved to be exactly what I had wanted. A small medical clinic housed in the office room was fully operational with the generous donations from Direct Relief International. Local workers would show up for treatment of conditions that varied from the removal of lumps and bumps to mastoiditis.

David Malalazi, an old friend and expert gardener, had come for several weeks to help us plant a medicinal garden around the house that included most of the healing plants of power. Along the road, we also planted large aloes harvested from the veld, which gave an elegant approach to the homestead. The garden had already been terraced and George had built small picturesque retaining walls with traditional Venda motifs where some of these plantings could be made.

One afternoon, after a heavy day of working with the tractor, George came into the clinic room where I was working with the plant database. He complained of pain in his chest on the left side at the back. He thought it had to do with sitting on the tractor all morning. His chest was clear when I listened with a stethoscope. The pain was aggravated by back movements and not deep breathing, so I presumed it was musculoskeletal rather than coming from his lungs. He had no fever. I gave him a strong anti-inflammatory analgesic. I was about to leave for the week and I expected to see him the following Monday after he came back from the weekend.

When I returned that Monday, Richard was there, but not George. I decided to wait until the next day before becoming concerned. By Tuesday George had still not shown up. I drove down to the village with Richard to find him. When we arrived at his house George came out and said that he had been sick but he had gone to see a *sangoma* who said he was bewitched. He had given him some medicine, amulets and a red cloth to wear around his neck for protection. He indicated that he was feeling much better and would be back to work in a day or two. He assured me that there was no need for me to examine him or worry about it. Richard and I took him at his word and drove back to *Tshisimane*. We were under constant attacks from witchcraft but, because of the protective *mutis*, this had never resulted in any sickness before.

Two days later George had still not shown up for work, so I drove back down to his house to check in. This time George did not come out of the house to greet me, and when I went in he looked terribly ill. He had a hacking cough with a fetid smell to it. I bundled him into the *bakkie* and drove him to the doctor in Makhado, who did an X-ray. She showed me the films that indicated that he had pneumonia in the left lung. She was also concerned about a lung abscess and suggested he be admitted to the local hospital for intravenous antibiotics. I took him in and consulted with the emergency room doctor, who transferred him to the ward in the care of another doctor. Meanwhile she began the treatment until the other doctor arrived. She said I should call the attending physician in the morning when he was available while doing ward rounds.

I knew this physician had a cell phone, but he would not give out the number. Communicating with the doctor was not as simple as she had made out. It seemed that the times he did his ward rounds were erratic or, alternatively, he did not feel the necessity to come to the phone and liaise with a colleague or return my calls. I did manage to get through to him on two occasions, but could hear that he resented my questions such as: "Did follow-up X-rays confirm there was an abscess?" (This would have considerably changed the length of time of antibiotic treatment and the prognosis.) "Were the tests for tuberculosis negative? And what was his HIV status?" He answered that there was no abscess, and everything had been negative for the other two. Intuitively I felt he did not really know the answers, even if the tests had indeed been done. When I asked about George's antibiotic coverage it was clear he was on an antiquated drug regime, probably a result of budget constraints and the fact that the public health system was largely dysfunctional. I thought George would need at least a week of intravenous antibiotics.

George called me the next day to come and fetch him, complaining that if I did not he would die there. I agreed that I could probably give him better care at *Tshisimane*. When I arrived, he said he was feeling much better, and stated he was scared to stay longer in case something bad happened to him. He said, "You remember the lump you removed from that worker's face that day and he was back at work the next day? Well there was another person with the same lump here, and after an operation he is still in the hospital a week later." Since he looked much better, I assumed he did not have a lung abscess and took him back to *Tshisimane* to convalesce.

I put him on a month of heavy-duty combination antibiotics since it was unlikely that a sputum culture had been done and any attempts to retrieve any results had been futile. I suspended him from work for at least six weeks and made sure that when I left he had nutritious food to eat and that Rupert would check in on him from time to time. I also gave him multivitamins to take to optimize his healing. When I returned the next time he told me that he had soon recovered completely.

After that our relationship shifted. When guests came they would tell me that George had told them how I had saved his life, and that he felt like my son. For the first time he began to ask me for divinations for some of his dilemmas, especially when his grandfather began to pressure him in his dreams to become initiated. We became friends rather than employer and employee, sharing dreams and deepening our relationship with the plants.

Apart from the groups and individuals that would come to experience *Tshisimane*, there was a steady flow of neighbors and also friends from inside and outside of South Africa who would come and stay for variable periods of time. However, there were occasions of a week or more where I was completely alone. I relished these times for creative work and reflection. Rupert and his family were welcome regulars, since they lived only 100 kilometers away. Rupert, being a tour guide and an excellent cook, was also an integral part of the program whenever we had a group from abroad coming for indigenous healing wisdom. These groups would spend a week at *Tshisimane* and then a further week traveling around Venda experiencing the culture, the wisdom of other *sangomas* and the excitement of the Kruger game reserve.

On one occasion I was expecting guests. I was driving back from Makhado that night and they were expected later. As I was approaching a nearby village an oncoming car began to flash its bright lights, partly blinding me. I suspected the driver thought that I had my brights on and he was telling me to dim them. I responded by flicking mine to show him otherwise, but he came back at me flashing his again. In the next instant I collided at 80 kilometers an hour with two cows. In an attempt to warn me, he had actually made it harder for me to see what was ahead. One cow was killed, and the other was paralyzed from a broken back.

The front of the *bakkie* was pushed in and battery acid was leaking out. An obliging Afrikaner family on their way to a party stopped to help. The driver dialed 911 while I dragged the cows off the road. The one that was paralyzed was flailing about helplessly with only its front legs, otherwise unable to move.

There are no fences in South Africa and accidents, including human fatalities, with animals are a frequent event, especially at night. I was not responsible for the cows being unattended, but I knew that if I hung around I would be confronted by someone demanding compensation, even though he may not even have been the owner of the animals. After 911 had been called and the animals were off the road, I decided to leave while my engine was still running. The helpful stranger was in agreement. He offered to put the paralyzed cow out of its misery with his firearm, but we both agreed this would not be a good idea. I was several miles away from the turnoff to *Tshisimane* and decided to try to get back as soon as possible, while the car was still running. I continued uneventfully until I reached the bottom of the mountain at Calitzdorp, where the engine and the entire electrical system died. I knew my guests would be along in an hour or two. I waited on the dirt road in the bush in the moonless night. Eventually I heard the sound of their Land Rover and got out to greet them.

Before I could say anything, they told me there had been an accident on the road. A police vehicle that had been called to the scene of an accident with two cows had hit another cow, which had totaled the police *bakkie*. My friends had experienced trouble getting past the carnage of three cows along the road and one battered police vehicle. I could not help myself from laughing out loud and then explaining why.

They drove up the hill and George came back down to fetch

me with the tractor. We hid the *bakkie* in the bush where Hendrik could not discover and strip it. George drove back up the mountain with me hanging onto the back of the tractor. By the time we reached the top, my hands had almost frozen to the metal. It was midwinter and very cold. We knew that Hendrik would have heard the tractor in the night and would be suspicious and come to investigate early the next morning. There was no time to lose, and after a few calls we went down the mountain early the next day to wait for the tow truck. The *bakkie* was hauled back to Makhado and in a week was fully repaired.

I was often surprised by the kind of service one could get in remote regions of South Africa. It rivaled that in the big cities and back home in California. I recall having a tooth abscess once and having a root canal treatment taken care of by a dentist in Polokwane. He had digital X-ray equipment that was more up to date than anything I had seen in Santa Barbara, and the excellent work he did was a fraction of the cost.

Whenever I went back to the USA, I was very fortunate that my friends Hannes and Marietjie, who owned the nearby Medike mountain lodge, made themselves available for support. Medike is a magnificent spot on the Sand River, with Bushman rock art and an unsurpassed canyon hike. Any visit there was enhanced by the wonderful warmth, cooking and hospitality of my friends. While I was away they would pay the salaries and attend to any matters that George could not cope with. Hannes was always happy to plug any gaps and include George's requests in his shopping lists. I could communicate with George if need be by phone, but also via email through Rupert or Medike. Much of the time the land-line at *Tshisimane* did not work. There was no cell signal on the mountain, so when the phone was not working George had to go down to where he could receive a signal and then call Rupert, who could email me about any emergencies, such as a fire that happened on one occasion. Fortunately, it was easily controlled and never got close to the homestead.

This system worked, but nevertheless the stress of maintaining a property on the opposite side of the world began to wear on me after a while. There was a constant drain on finances, which was only partially covered by donations and the revenues from groups. This later made it much easier for me to ultimately resign myself to giving in to the land claims that surfaced.

My friend Peter, who worked high up in government circles in nearby Waterberg, gave me sobering advice when he said, "Dave, it will not be long before you will be old and maybe not fit enough to travel a long distance, work so hard, and even walk these mountains anymore—then this place will be too much for you. Find yourself something more practical." My attorney in Makhado had similar advice: "Dave, you cannot have two homes! It just will not work!"

I knew the ancestors tolerated my African dream, but were only truly supportive of the deepening of my healing skills, and not necessarily anything else unrelated. They warned:

*Are you nibbling on the apples of the Tree of Knowledge
or are you nurturing whatever proud plant or
humble weed is your present entrustment?
It is that which you are to make glorious.*

My proud plant or humble weed was healing, rather than any of my building, gardening or managerial projects. The ancestors had always made clear that my job was to take from South Africa to bring to the USA, not the other way around.

I was to help introduce African healing wisdom to the West.

My surgical mentor, Professor Duplessis, would say to us regarding a particular, possibly unnecessary, proposed surgery, "Is this journey really necessary?" My ancestors, always making allowances for free will, were wondering the same. I realized that much of my journey at *Tshisimane* was about fulfilling a dream to have my own place in the African bush. The rest was about learning more about indigenous healing wisdom. It was only the latter that they wanted to favor. Furthermore, early on during my *Thwasa*, my grandfather had come to Maryellen in a dream and said, "Tell David that he is the healing center, he does not need a place!"

The ancestors, harping on one's destiny, would reiterate:

Anything that does not make you more of who you are,
makes you less of who you are.

Look carefully to what you aspire, cherish and guard so
as not to squander your gifts nor lose your heritage.

Being aware of the lesson is different from learning it.
Knowing the path is different from following it.

Such were the trials and tribulations from some of the worst troublemakers during my stay. Some others, not mentioned here, will appear in the subsequent chapter on witchcraft.

This takes me back to my original visit when I first bought *Tshisimane*. I had seen an exquisite red duiker standing sentinel on the road near the roofless homestead. This boded well for much light in the future for the center. On the other hand, when Rupert and I exited the property and stopped to visit the exquisite riverine area with its pool, we had also seen two black mambas. This message was a prophecy about the darker aspects of the challenges we were still to face.

In retrospect, if I had known what was to happen, would I have purchased the land? Absolutely and unequivocally yes. The light far outweighed the dark at the end of the day.

XV

The Groups

INWARD BOUND WAS ESTABLISHED IN 1995, AND UNTIL I developed *Tshisimane* we had been taking trips to Peru, the Kalahari, the Sinai, and then more recently to Limpopo. However, once I was initiated as a *sangoma*, the tools I had for inner healing expanded significantly. *Tshisimane* was ideal, not only for the Inward Bound journey, but also to immerse participants in the magic of indigenous healing wisdom. The format now changed somewhat, since I had dedicated the place to suit the needs for both experiences. The two were complementary. The Garden of Eden archetype not only was necessary for Inward Bound, but was also essential for the best *sangoma* medicine.

I brought groups to *Tshisimane* to allow them to experience the magic of Africa, walk in the bush and connect with the trees and plants, the birds and the wildlife. In addition, yoga, meditations, bone divinations and appropriate rituals were provided to help them on their transpersonal journeys. We made appropriate use of the labyrinth and the Native American Medicine Wheel that also speaks so profoundly to the power of the four directions in nature. Every day we would have a council or talking circle where dreams and experiences were shared. These had always been part of Inward Bound's programs. Now plants for dreaming were readily available and could be used accordingly. Individuals would also have divinations, followed up with medicines and rituals depending on their individual readings. Healing baths with appropriate plants were also dispensed for various psycho-spiritual dysfunctions.

It was stressed that when it came to delving into our own intuitive work it was vital that each one of us realize that we have our own specific avenue of communication that we should nurture. We should not look at the gifts others have and be discouraged by our lack of them. There were many ways we could acknowledge spirit input, such as a buzzing in the ear, muscles twitching in the shoulder, or a tingling up the spine. Even those that were good dreamers needed some help in remembering their dreams, which were frequently scripted by the ancestors. Participants were reassured that they should not necessarily expect to hear voices or have visions, but that they might have bodily sensations that told them what feels right and what feels wrong. A gut feeling may inform us that something is amiss, and if we experience goose bumps it may be that a profound inner truth has just been revealed or acknowledged. Others just had a deep internal sense of "knowing." Nature lovers might see signs in nature that could come as metaphors carried by the wind, an animal, a bird or the glow of a sunset. Animals could present themselves in and outside of dreams. The ancestors might guide these animals to us when we need help.

There would usually be one or two groups per year from abroad, and visitors that would come up from different parts of Southern Africa, especially from Johannesburg. Group process was based around the concept of the archetypal journey of the hero. In The Hero With a Thousand Faces Joseph Campbell says, "The hero ventures forth from the world of common day into a region of supernatural wonder. Fabulous forces are there encountered and a decisive victory is won. The hero comes back from this mysterious adventure with the power to bestow boons on his fellow man."

In the traditional concept of *Thwasa*, the initiation process of the *sangoma*, the initiate is undergoing a hero's journey similar to the Venda youth undergoing his circumcision and initiation into adulthood. *Thwasa* is the process of maturation in which the "new moon develops into a full moon."

These examples are typical of archetypal phenomena. The different themes are all similar in principle. The journey of the hero or heroine, the journey of initiation and any rite of passage, have been defined by Arnold Van Genet as occurring in three distinct phases: severance or separation, threshold or the journey itself, and incorporation or integration. The hero's journey is the quest for one's own higher Self, a journey into one's own psyche. It is also a person's search for his or her own individual destiny. If at all possible, it would be best to find it this lifetime rather than in future ones. In the words of one of my dream songs, I sang to myself, "Oh please don't let me take this trip again."

In the first phase of separation the hero hears the call to adventure. He or she must either follow it or smother something within. This call is a yearning for the extraordinary. The first level of resistance must be overcome – usually work, home, spouse, children, friends, etc. telling him or her not to go.

The judgment of the 99 neither validates nor
invalidates the worth of the one. The many and the few
do not speak to value, only to popularity.
Popularity is not to be equated with value.

Once "separated," guides assist the hero to point out the

dangers and show the way. This is the phase where synchronicity may appear. Jung described synchronicity as a meaningful coincidence where two events occur simultaneously, linking the inner psyche with an outer event. For example, one makes a decision to take a trip and information arrives that day describing the very trek you wish to take. The hero may be armed or given a symbol of power, such as a sword in the classical tales of old. Today this is more likely to be some form of knowledge in the form of a book or a teacher to help one on the way.

Following separation, the hero enters into the second phase: the threshold or the journey itself. Archetypically this takes place in nature, in wilderness, a cave or a forest. The hero passes into a world of supernatural wonder where strange forces are encountered and the ordinary world is left behind. An obstacle or physical force is met, such as a dragon, guard, or fierce dog, which must be overcome before victory is won. The hero/ine faces death and physical danger before encountering the dangers of the psyche, the shadow parts of his/her life, or the dark night of the soul. This is critical for the hero to be reborn, or become whole, self-actualized and self-realized. With the knowledge and confidence of the success of the first physical obstacle, and with the object of power, the hero is able to overcome the more difficult second confrontation, the struggle with his basic fear. Of the two fears, the psychological can be greater than the physical. Having prevailed, the hero earns the reward of a grail and the treasure of inner knowledge. With this new gift, the magical numinous world can be left behind. The hero departs the threshold with a new awareness and returns home with knowledge and power to help or heal.

Now the phase of incorporation begins. The journey cannot be completed unless the hero brings the wisdom of the experience back to the community. The whole journey is ultimately an altruistic one. During the phases of separation and threshold fear will come up with all its manifestations. Without confronting fear, the archetypal journey of the hero cannot be fulfilled.

In my case the instrument of power for separation had been the vivid dream of *Tshisimane's* landscape. This was followed by the trials, tribulations and significant dangers of developing an indigenous healing center on the top of a mountain with very poor access and a lot of local opposition (threshold phase). The incorporation, on my return to California, was the opportunity to use all the knowledge I had gleaned on the journey.

Our true destiny is usually bound up in some way with a hero or heroine's journey or journeys. There are fewer heroes in public life these days. While many people complete the first two phases, few complete the third phase of incorporation. An example of this is the Olympic athlete who fulfills the phases of separation and threshold. However, the phase of incorporation, where something is taken back to the community, is often lacking. Without the incorporation of the gifts back into society, their particular journey is more accurately termed the "warrior's journey." Our Western society is replete with successful warriors.

So-called "primitive" peoples seem to understand the psychological importance of the process and use it to the greatest effect to make their young men whole. At a certain age they are forcibly "separated" from their mothers and the womenfolk to undergo rigorous training with the older men, finally culminating in a terrifying ordeal such as ritual circumcision. After this they can integrate back into the tribe or group as men and take on new responsibilities. Today, among many African tribes, this rite of passage is still intact, and ritual circumcision is a significant part of it. Hunting of an animal may be another part of the process. In the case of the Masai, the hunting of a lion was required, but today is not permitted. Through these types of challenges and accomplishments, the three phases of initiation are fulfilled.

The psychological and physical pain a boy must endure in some cultures, with surgical removal of his foreskin without anesthesia or even a sharp scalpel, is something few of his counterparts in the Western world would be able to endure. Venda girls undergo their own initiation, culminating in the amazing spectacle of the *Domba* or python dance. At the end of an intense period of initiation, hundreds of young women, naked from the waist up, form a sinuous, dancing chain which simulates the movement of a huge python. The *Domba* is not only a python dance but is also symbolic of fertility and of how the fetus moves in the uterus. The Venda, like most Southern African tribes, believe in the *Kundalini*-like concept of a primal snake that rests in the lower belly which is feminine and is key not only to fertility, but also to spiritual power. It is responsible for the release of the ova and is also thought to control the whole body. During the initiation process, of which the dance is a part, the initiates are taught sex education and are made powerful and fit not only by vigorous dancing but also by repetitive squatting and crouching to make them strong for labor and delivery. They also have to fetch heavy containers of water carried on their heads from the river.

For a Westerner, a struggle with an illness such as breast cancer can easily take on the dimensions of the heroine's journey. There are other parallels as well. In indigenous cultures the elders of the society are in attendance to support and validate the ordeal. The youth will carry this experience all of his or her life, and retrieve it from the psyche when the need for strength, courage and fortitude arise. Armed with this past experience, the initiate can believe in his ability to handle whatever comes his way. I cannot help but think that this inner strength has enabled many Africans to endure, with equanimity and courage, the numerous trials and tribulations the continent continuously offers up to them.

At *Tshisimane* we designed the experience to fit the three phases first described by Van Gennep. In the first phase of severance, we separated from past conditioning and old patterns of behavior. We dropped away from our stereotypes of teacher, nurse, lawyer, engineer or doctor so that we could reach into something fresh and new about ourselves. With an open, empty mind, not filled or restricted by stale conditioning, we were more able to receive what the sacred space of *Tshisimane* had to offer. Some considered changing their name for the duration of the trip.

During the threshold phase, emotional baggage would come up as a manifestation of another archetype, the shadow, where we projected our dark side onto others in the form of judgment and blame. A forum for expressing feelings was offered in the talking circle, and this helped defuse touchy situations. An outlet for some of the powerful emotions that surfaced was provided, but participants had to take responsibility for their own journey, both physical and spiritual. In circle we were only allowed to discuss our own feelings. No finger pointing was permitted.

Finally, at the end of the journey, the group entered the

phase of incorporation or integration, when reentry depression could occur. The "departure" from wilderness was designed to be mindful and the reentry was discussed so that participants were prepared for some strong emotions, both positive and negative. Very often the group only realized how profound the effect had been during the re-entry phase. On their return others they encountered now seemed strange, and there was a general feeling of sensory overload. This was often the first inkling to the seeker that they had in fact been in an altered state of consciousness and experiencing wilderness rapture. The inward aspects of the trip were best kept to oneself upon return because they could be misunderstood. The outward components were more easily described and less likely to lead to discord back home. Participants were discouraged from making any major life changes until these powerful effects had subsided several weeks later. The subconscious and spiritual effect of the trip could continue to work for many months and manifested itself in different ways, including major lifestyle changes.

The "real you" was likely to be the primal you, out in the wild, the one more deeply connected with your inner being. When readapted to the various toxicities that society imposed, this "you" was often supplanted by a persona-like version of the original. We needed to remember who we truly were. If we could not permanently carry this back, we at least needed to reconnect with it from time to time by making contact with the Higher Self through some form of spiritual practice.

Everyone was encouraged to continue practices that had been introduced on the trip, such as breath work, meditation and yoga. This needed to be enjoyable and sustainable, done for its own sake and without any agenda or goal. The overwhelming overload of external stimuli and food for the ego could tend to suck us back into former ways of being and old patterns. A regular connection with some form of inner discipline could prevent this. Connecting with others made reentry easier – group energy was generally self-supporting and powerful.

The hero could return with a profound vision or more often just a sense of clarity as to how to be better in the world. This sometimes translated itself into doing one's existing job with more compassion and intensity, and not necessarily making dramatic changes in one's life. We could either change what we were doing or change the way in which we did it. The same was true for relationships that could either be given up or negotiated in a different way. A regular practice and group participation could prevent the "fall," or the sacrifice of the rediscovered Self to material pursuits.

Managing the reentry or incorporation phase was summarized to our groups as follows:

1. Acknowledge the reentry depression as a gift resulting from a profound encounter with your true Self. It is an indicator of the intensity of the wilderness rapture and the prior altered state of consciousness. Sometimes the more powerful the journey, the more the temporary depression.

2. Separate needs from wants on the return. It is the "want" and not the "need" that can sabotage a successful integration. Beware the seduction of materialism. There is nothing wrong with material things as long as the energy required to sustain them does not take you

away from "following your bliss." It is fine to have good things, but not okay if they have you.

3. Practice the walk and suppress the talk. Live the vision rather than describe it. Family and friends are more likely to pay attention to a shift in behavior for the better than to any transformational experience described in words.

4. Do not dive back into old habits and addictions. Substitute a form of spiritual practice that is enjoyable, practical and likely to last. One cannot face the challenges of modern society without the help of some method of going inward. This does not have to be anything esoteric; surfing can be more powerful than meditation, gardening as good as Tai Chi.

5. Develop a community that can be self-supporting. There can be a synergy in groups.

6. As Joseph Campbell teaches, live out your vision, be true to your own myth, and follow your bliss.

Listen to the heart's whisper. Within our deepest Self are thoughts that are not spoken and feelings that are not expressed because of our timidity of their reception. Deep Self is where the soul dwells so if you ever hear their cries or feel their stirrings, risk ridicule of any sort for your very soul could be in danger of erosion.
When the heart is muffled, the soul shrinks.

The essence of incorporation was to give the gift gained from the journey away. This act would bring just as many benefits to the giver as it would to the receiver.

"I don't know what your destiny will be, but one thing I do know, the only ones among you who will be really happy are those who have sought and found how to serve."
Albert Schweitzer

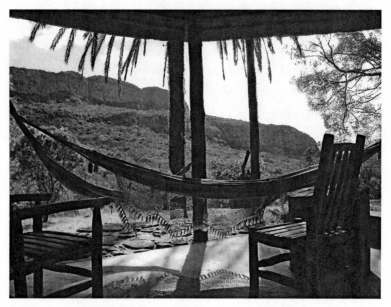

Meditative mountain view from the porch

XVI

witchcraft, sorcery and such

We have a dark and a light side to our nature. The dark side of our nature must be properly confronted – neither dismissed nor conquered but acknowledged for what it is, even valued as such.

To make a choice, good and evil must both operate freely. The only way to do away with evil is to continually choose the good. Evil is not the cause, but rather the consequence, of not choosing God's revealed will. This is what gives it birth and sustains its life.

When we choose God's revealed will, the consequence is good.

This too is what gives goodness its birth and sustains life. It is important to understand that it is neither evil nor good that cause our choice but rather that they are theconsequence of it.

Free will is always neutral, motivated and catalyzed by desire.

You cannot say, "the devil made me do it."

BEFORE MOVING ON TO THE NEXT SECTION ON WITCHES, I should make clear that the word "witch" has two polarities in Western understanding: good and bad. There are light witches and dark witches. The stories here relate only to witches that work on the dark side. The white witches are best associated with what is called Wicca in the West. In Southern Africa the term "witch" usually refers to someone working on the dark side. In Zulu the word for witch is *"umthakati."*

Unfortunately, it is true to say that not all *sangomas* work on behalf of the light. I was very fortunate in having P.H. Mntshali and later Andries as my teachers, both of whom were very firm in their integrity and impeccable in relationship to the ancestors. P.H. always warned that if one did not remain true to the healing, the ancestors would leave and the *sangoma* would then have no power. If this happened it could sometimes result in a *sangoma* resorting to trickery, or possibly signing on with dark spirits and becoming a witch.

Witchcraft arises from a heart of envy and jealousy. This speaks to one of the Ten Commandments that prohibits covetousness:

"You shall not covet your neighbor's house; you shall not covet your neighbor's wife or his male servant or his female servant or his ox or his donkey or anything that belongs to your neighbor." Exodus 20:17

Witchcraft from this side of the veil can deprive one of choice. The malicious intent is to control, often for demonic, usually destructive and always self-serving purposes.

david cumes, md

When their power seems ineffective with someone, they will frequently take out their frustration in both physical and emotional harassment that demoralize, thus impairing any effectiveness for good.

I was once walking in the bush with a Tsonga tracker in the Kruger area looking for medicinal plants and we were talking about this. His description of what can happen haunts me. It went like this.

"Anyone can get this power to be a witch. All you have to do is go to a powerful witch and ask him or her. He or she will sell you a 'snake' that can then bring you anything you need. But you will have to 'feed' your snake forever. If you eat, he must eat. You must share your profits with him. If you stop feeding him he will get angry and then he will begin to eat your wife, your children, your family. You get power and money, but you are a slave to your snake."

This story instructs us as to what happens when one engages a powerful evil spirit to do your bidding. The price one pays is the cost of your soul.

The witches and sorcerers whose revenue comes from creating hurt and harm are the opposite polarity to the *sangoma*'s healing arts. Unfortunately, among white people in Southern Africa, this group has sometimes been included into the now mixed-bag title of "*sangoma*." This may have occurred due to apartheid, which led to poor understanding as to the sophistication of Bantu cultures' spirit medicine. The "Witchcraft Act," instituted years previously by the British, was an attempt to stop witchcraft. As any *sangoma* will tell you, it is impossible to stop witchcraft. It is part of God's creation: no light without dark. It is up to us to choose light. All the Act did was to push witchcraft further underground. Witches prefer that no one know they are witches so they can ply their trade without opposition. Furthermore, if people are ignorant of their power, this is to the witches' advantage.

The most clever and insidious achievement of the dark
forces is in making some people disbelieve
in their existence.

Many whites growing up in apartheid South Africa believed that light and dark were more or less inseparably linked in anyone practicing as a *sangoma* or *nyanga*. This belief, as well as the blatant misconception that the Bantu were heathens who did not believe in God, was for obvious reasons reinforced by the missionaries and the church.

Witchcraft tends to be a lucrative profession since one can charge huge prices to bewitch someone's opposition in business or possibly even a husband so that the client could solicit the favors of the man's wife. For the right price, a victim could even be killed by a witch's hex or a sorcerer's poison. Furthermore, there was not necessarily direct cause and effect, and a spell that was cast could take time to work. This added to Western skepticism as to the effectiveness of this malevolent skill.

There is no temporal relationship when intention is
activated, whether it be light or dark. When healing or
harming is set in place, the result
may take time to evolve.

Early on in my *sangoma* initiation, like most white South Africans, I did not believe witchcraft had any power unless the person who was bewitched knew they had been hexed and be-lieved in it. In other words the nocebo response, or the ability of belief to harm, hurt or kill, was responsible for the dam-age caused. The more the fear, I thought, the more the power of nocebo, whereas its opposite, profound healing, is invoked with the magic of love.

Fear can be a friend if it alerts and warns. It is a magician in conjuring up all manner of images. Whatever we do not reason with or dismiss becomes its own reality. Fear conquers when we let its possibilities project as realities directing and controlling our actions and decisions.

Fear itself is not a foe, but acquiescing to fear empowers it to be a formidable one.

After my initiation I learned that witchcraft can create harm regardless of whether the individual believes in or knows about the spell. I began to understand why there is a com-mandment that tells us not to be envious or jealous. If someone covets something, apart from stealing it or murdering for it, the next step might be to go to a witch or a sorcerer and make a re-quest to possess that thing that belongs to someone else. In the West some people use dishonest lawyers for this; in indigenous cultures they use witchcraft.

If we ignore or discount the very real and constant threat of negative forces, we do so at our peril.

Depending on the power of the sorcerer, the spell can be very effective, even causing fatalities. Many of us growing up in

South Africa were familiar with at least one story of a black person who had been bewitched who had gone home to die, believing that the spell was so powerful it could not be reversed. Any spell associated with guilt on the part of the victim has far more power, and this factor may have been operative in these dramatic instances. Theoretically, it should always be possible to find a *sangoma* who has more powerful ancestors than the witch's evil spirits, enabling him or her to reverse the curse.

Sangomas who work with less pure spirits and who do not heal consistently also exist. For what they consider the right reason or price, they might, on occasion, practice witchcraft. There are also tricksters who appear to be *sangomas*, but who are actually primarily witches or sorcerers. It is this principle that probably makes it difficult for *sangomas* to share their knowledge openly, because one never knows who is a witch, or who might become one. *Sangomas* have warned me to be wary of a witch masquerading as a client or patient. I have known instances of *sangomas*, and curanderos in Peru, who started off as excellent healers but because of material temptations "turned" to the dark side.

> *The dark forces use water to cool our desire to do good*
> *and fire to heat our desire to do wrong, while the forces*
> *of light use water to cool our desire to do wrong and fire*
> *to heat our desire to do good. And so it is we must look to*
> *our intent, for it is that which dictates*
> *the uses of fire and water.*

The witch prefers to be "the traitor within the gates," a person who would rather not be known to be a witch, so that he or she can continue to practice unopposed. *Sangomas* have told me that, from time to time, they have been consulted professionally by witches who would come to test their power, or try to learn some of their secrets or medicines. Any knowledge shared could then be turned against the *sangoma*. Persons who are powerful advocates for the light are always at risk. Moreover, witches may seek to test their own dark power against that of the ancestors working on the *sangoma's* behalf. The paradigm is much like cowboy history and "the fastest gun in the West." If you are powerful, others will come looking for you to see if they are better. Witches are even competitive and adversarial amongst one another.

Those that have many guides, and are greatly beloved,
will have many dissuaders and be greatly envied.

It is also important for Westerners to realize that witchcraft can be quite subtle rather than dramatic and bizarre. It may manifest as a black mamba that has been energetically manipulated to wait for you on your path. It may also present as anxiety, depression, bad luck and strange dynamics arising among family and loved ones, creating divorce, substance abuse and other maladies that otherwise might be logically assigned to other causes.

When I first decided to get initiated in Swaziland, what I really wanted to do was use the diagnostic magic of the bones to help counsel people. What I did not fully appreciate was that helping people was also going to involve counteracting negative energies that impacted the patient's well-being, such as intrusive spirits, energetic pollution, witchcraft and sorcery. When I first discussed this with P.H. in Swaziland I said to him, "Well, I do not want to be dealing with that stuff. I do not particularly enjoy being involved with negative forces." He would smile and say, "You will be dealing with this whether you like it or not."

Just prior to having our book on medicinal trees and plants of the Lowveld published, I gave a promotional talk with Rael Loon, a coauthor, to some of the Big Five private game lodges in the southern part of the Kruger National Park. These are five-star retreats where local visitors, and more especially those from abroad, come to view game in open vehicles with experienced game guides. Our idea was to go to the game guides and promote the book to them as a resource for their guests who were also interested in African lore and the various uses of medicinal plants in this unique Lowveld ecosystem. The guides were already quite familiar with much of the information, but we thought that a small handbook on the subject would help to amplify their knowledge. To promote the book, we offered a presentation focusing on the uses of the plants of power, especially by the Venda and the Tsonga peoples. One of the questions I posed to the guides, half of whom were black, was, "Who here believes that witchcraft only works if you believe that it will work?" All the white game guides put up their hands, but none of the black game guides did. I was somewhat surprised that even these white guides who were so steeped in the knowledge of bush lore were misinformed. They went along with the common misconception in South Africa, among whites, that witchcraft only works against black people because they believe in it. This could not be further from the truth. I gave some of the examples from my own experience, and later on one of the black game guides came up to me and joked, "But now you are telling them all of our secrets."

If one has a strong belief in witchcraft and this is combined with the effect of the hex itself, this can be even more harmful. These two factors of hexing plus nocebo account for the seeming discrepancy in the effect witchcraft has on whites versus blacks. The fact that one does not believe in witchcraft does not make one immune to its effects, but an additional strong belief in it will magnify the power. Guilt will further enhance its manifestation, so that if one has done something wrong, and has been bewitched as retribution, the curse may have more impetus. This may be because, at a conscious or subconscious level, the victim feels they deserve to succumb or be punished.

Sometimes I believe that one of the reasons I ended up at *Tshisimane* in the heart of Venda is because Venda is known to have many witches and sorcerers skilled in their dark craft. My ancestors wanted to impress upon me the importance of this power wherever we may live, since witchcraft is ubiquitous. The witches in Venda are renowned for their expertise in spells, potions and poisons. When I first met Andries he said to me, "Do not go and visit the *sangomas* in the Venda villages and spend time with them, because many deal too much in witchcraft." I took his advice.

I was aware of the fact that witches could place medicine along the path and at the front of the door of your house, and if you walked across this you could get extremely ill and even die. This is called *"tshifula"* in Venda. George confirmed that even though white people do not believe in witchcraft it can affect them in certain ways that they would not recognize, such as bad luck, or even one's car mysteriously going off the road, resulting in an accident.

Kabbalah discourses on the evil eye, the evil tongue, the evil inclination, and the evil wind or spirit. *Sangoma* wisdom would go along with these principles. The evil eye is a form of negativity in which one might sense being "bad vibed." It does not feel good, but may not always be particularly harmful. However, if a person has a lot of "magical power" and someone has done something harmful to him or her, the evil eye can sometimes cause serious damage. The story of Willem demonstrates this possibility. This was also the "final straw" of thatch that occurred with Willem the roofer.

The ongoing problems with the leaking house roof continued. In spite of all the roof issues and his violent temper, Willem was a relatively likable, charismatic character and I enjoyed his company when he came periodically to inspect his work and give further instructions. He would bring his crew from Polokwane for more than a week at a time and usually left them with enough supplies for the job and food for the stay.

I wanted to be sure the roof was corrected before the expiration date of the five-year guarantee. However, there was little incentive for Willem, who was a trickster, to come all the way out to patch something under guarantee. I would stimulate him with further projects so that he could justify the cost of his coming, and patch the roof at the same time. His bookkeepers were his wife and daughter whom, I learned, ran a tight ship while Willem practiced his craft. I assumed that their insistence on a high profit margin had something to do with his periodic nasty changes in behavior. Hence he tried all the tricks he knew, short of doing a major reconstruction which would cost him money, to stop the roof leaks. The chimney continued to be a source of leakage in spite of redoing the concrete and the flashing around it several times. When it rained we became used to a wet floor in the kitchen and living-dining area. There were no carpets to ruin and the water rapidly dried up, but this did not make me feel better about the leaky roof. Willem wore less and less well with time, especially when it came to his workers, who though extremely skilled and always helpful, I suspected were underpaid.

The east side of the house, the outside bathrooms, the lapa and the healing hut were spaced about a hundred yards apart, more or less in a straight line running east. There was a magnificent buttress of rocks between the bathrooms and the lapa. For some time I had thought of making a rustic bedroom for myself in this special place that looked out directly north onto the spectacular mountain ridge, and Willem was now erecting a thatch roof around the rock feature. The roof design for the new hut was simple, and Willem had left the workers with building materials, some supplies and food to continue. The workers were always accommodated and fed in George's living space. This time they not only ran out of food, which we then provided, but they also ran out of building materials. A spectacular thatch roof, however, was mostly completed over the rock formation that was to form the western wall of the room.

Willem came a week later than he was supposed to and, being out of materials and unable to work, some of the workers had walked down to the village below out of frustration and boredom. When he arrived to find this he was furious, even more so because the workers had improved on the roof design so that it better fit the rock feature. They had thought that this must obviously have been Willem's intent, since it was logical. Willem deduced from this that he would now have to bring more thatch than he had budgeted for, and he threatened to make them tear it down and do it again the way he said he had told them in the beginning. This certainly had not been clear to me, nor to them, and the design they had made was entirely correct. He also said that since they had messed up, he would not pay them to do any of this additional remedial work. I intervened and told Willem they had done a great job and it should be left as it was, and that I would absorb any additional cost for the thatch. This was all done with much yelling and screaming by him while the workers listened quietly. No mention was made of the fact that they had not been given enough food or any wages, and had been idle for days waiting for Willem to arrive on schedule.

> *Words have great power. They acknowledge, affirm and*
> *inspire. They strengthen, heal and comfort.*
> *They express intention, love and gratitude.*
> *They are messengers of laughter.*

But the opposite can also have a consequence.

After his tirade, Willem took off in a rage in his 4x4 *bakkie* to go back to Polokwane, and George and I took my *bakkie* into the bush to look for medicines. It was not long before we heard a tractor driving down the mountain, and George recognized from its sound that it was ours. Neither of us could come to any other conclusion but that our tractor was being stolen. I raced on after it, having to reach the road through the thick bush first, which gave the criminal a head start. We eventually saw the tractor racing at full speed down the treacherous road. Three of Willem's workers were hanging onto it, including the driver, who was doing an excellent job on the challenging curves and corrugated, potted dirt road. We all arrived simultaneously at a spot where we found an irate Willem standing impatiently in the middle of the road, hands on hips, apparently without his *bakkie*. When we looked more closely, we saw the *bakkie* perched on a tree that kept it from falling far down into the canyon below. Willem's steering linkage had come apart and, if not for the tree, he, his passenger and his *bakkie* would have come to an unfortunate end. They had both climbed out and up the ravine, and Willem had sent his passenger running back to fetch the tractor. We had not been around to ask, and so one of his workers had done the obvious thing. He knew tractors well and, with a few other workers, had taken it down the mountain to rescue his boss. This did not prevent Willem from excoriating him because he had not asked my permission. We pulled the vehicle out with the tractor, and Willem fixed the linkage adequately enough to limp home. I am sure the workers smiled and joked on their way back to the homestead.

I have no proof that the evil eye or even a possible evil inclination had anything to do with this nearly fatal event. However, the way George and my eyes met when we saw what had happened certainly confirmed to both of us that this may have been no accident. There is no question that the evil eye can have power, though some might prefer to say, "What goes around, comes around." This cliché recognizes a phenomenon that has been around since the beginning of time.

This also proved to be the closing event in the relationship between *Tshisimane* and Willem. After realizing he could not make enough profit on a floor he had begun for the same hut, he walked off the job and refused to come back and honor the guarantee on the roof. At the end of this saga the workers had the last word, leaving a telling symbol of the great job they had done on the roof. On my next visit back, I noted a huge and magnificent tobacco plant growing tall next to the hut, probably from one of the seeds that dropped from one of the roofer's tobacco. Tobacco is a traditional offering used to greet and thank the ancestors.

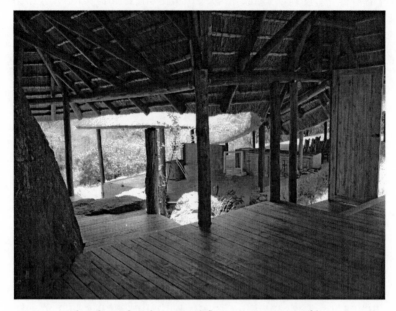

Thatch roof and eventual floor construction of hut

The evil tongue, another facet of witchcraft, is around us constantly, especially in the media, where people are frequently being character assassinated and have a lot of difficulty recovering from accusations that may not be true. The evil tongue is a vile form of negativity that can destroy a person's life. Even idle gossip can be harmful.

An evil inclination may compel a person who only seeks to do ill, and this is germane to witches and sorcerers. Once the evil inclination of a witch combines with a malevolent spirit who also seeks to do harm, much damage can ensue. This was true for the witches in the villages down at the bottom of *Tshisimane* mountain, and a white *sangoma* in the process of building a healing center would be a preferred target for their antics. George said to me quite early on when we met, "They will come and visit you at night," and this proved to be true.

david cumes, md

*Some living persons, through deliberate intensely
concentrated energy focus, can influence, trigger and
even sometimes invade another's dream realm.*

On one occasion I remember sleeping in my bed and literally
being almost thrown out of it by some energetic force. This was
not a nightmare – it was real. If it had happened in California I
might have thought it was an earthquake. When I told George
about it he said, "It's witchcraft; let's go and see Andries and see
what he has to say." Andries confirmed the fact that they had been
attempting to discourage and maybe even kill me, and he used the
word "tilo," which in Shangaan means "lightning." Lightning is a
particularly malevolent form of witchcraft in which powerful sorcerers and witches are said to be able to even manipulate lightning
to eliminate you or your homestead. Among the Zulus, a bird
called a *Hammerkop* (*impundulu* or lightning bird) is supposed to
be sent by witches as the carrier of this bolt of lightning. It could
be energetic as in my case, but sometimes possibly could also be
literal. Andries reassured me that my ancestors were powerful and
had protected me from harm.

*If you walk with your ancestors you will take an abundance
of powerful forces with you. They will dispel, neutralize, shed
and shade the negative ones that await.
The closer those that are spiritually powerful get to the Light,
the more likely will there be negative forces also of great
power to deter them.
The power of a spiritual gift is a challenge to them.
Your spirit guides will be there for support, to give their own
blessing and also to keep the dark forces away.*

Sangomas believe that dreaming or seeing a black or green mamba is a warning that danger may be pending. The color green is associated with envy, and I have been warned more than once by a green mamba dream.

On one occasion I had invited a prominent *sangoma* to introduce my book, Africa in my Bones, at the book launch in Johannesburg. The night after calling and asking him, I dreamed I was at *Tshisimane* and a large green mamba slithered down the chimney and attempted to attack me in spite of the fact that I was backing away. It struck at me and, just in time, an invisible hand grabbed it before it could sink its fangs into my arm. I called him to cancel my invitation, telling his receptionist that my ancestors had appeared to me in a dream and told me to invite someone else. She took no issue with any instructions coming from the ancestral realm and told me she would relay the message. I later confirmed that this *sangoma* was known to be envious and to sometimes work on the dark side. I also recalled him asking me why his name was not acknowledged in the book and why he was not sharing in the royalties.

The appearance of a python in dreams or in the waking state is an endorsement by the ancestors and is a sign that they are in agreement with what you are doing. It is a confirmation of spiritual empowerment. Not surprisingly, therefore, George had wanted to catch one and put it in the *ndumba* healing hut to help our visitors dream better.

I have been able to extend these same lessons to snakes in California. A rattlesnake is usually a warning to me of some sort, and the colorful benign king snake a message of support. On one occasion a friend and I were on a backpacking trip in the southern California desert when we saw a rattlesnake behaving in an unusual way. It seemed unafraid, did not rattle, and slid alongside only a few yards away and parallel to us for several minutes before it headed off into the desert. It was also an unusual, reddish "danger" color. We had found no water where we had planned our hike and were thinking about diverting to an alternative trail. The rattlesnake was enough to make me rethink this idea and we headed back to Santa Barbara after spending a night in the mountains en route. Later on we learned that not only was there no water anywhere else, but also that severe fires around San Diego had caused the roads to be closed, and that we would have been stuck there for days if we had not left when we did.

During the years I spent at *Tshisimane* reviewing all the books on medicinal plants, one book in particular spoke about the different forms of witchcraft and the medicines used for it in Zimbabwe. It cited specific potions that could be laid across one's path, and those used for poisoning food, that could both create a lingering painful illness. It seemed to me unscientific to expect that a sickness could be caused just by walking over an area where a curse had been placed. I rationalized that what really happened was that the medicine was impregnated on thorns that could impale someone walking along the path, especially if they were barefoot. Until relatively recently most people in rural areas walked barefoot. These bizarre illnesses could only be recognized and countered by an experienced *sangoma*. It was diabolical that shortly after that book had been published, the author, an M.D., mysteriously died.

A friend of mine had experienced this very thing and it had taken her months to get well. She related that one day she had sat in her usual place in her hut and had leaned up against the wall – a wall made of adobe, with a roof of thatch. She became aware of being pricked by a thorn that had been cleverly planted where she was known to always sit. This led to months of a debilitating illness that traveled throughout her body and manifested in different ways with diverse symptoms of malaise, fever, weakness, body aches and abdominal pains which Western doctors were unable to diagnose. She recognized the symptoms, understood what had happened, and was able to find an old *sangoma* knowledgeable about this form of sorcery. Over a period of months he managed to counteract it.

Andries had already protected my 4x4 when I first purchased it, and this particular 1987 Toyota was one of the best models ever made. It was reputed to be one of the most stolen cars in Southern Africa. The engine was extremely durable and was often removed and placed in one of the ubiquitous taxis seen on the roads. The fact that my vehicle was never stolen or tampered with, in spite of having no other security system and mostly was unlocked, was a testament to the power of Andries' ancestors and his "medicine." When I finally gave the pickup to George, before I left *Tshisimane*, he asked me to protect it for him, correctly stating that the medicine needed to be renewed now that he was the owner. I spent several hours protecting it but had forgotten all about it until one day when we visited Andries who was there at his gate to greet us as we drove up. Without him even knowing about what I had done, he looked at the car and said to George in Shangaan, "Dave did a good job of protecting the car." In some way he was able to "see" it. I was astonished.

When I first arrived at *Tshisimane* and the land claims surfaced, we came into contact with Silas, a particularly nasty person, who headed up the claim for the claimant group that he represented and was also part of. Silas started off benignly enough. When I first bought the property, he would call Rupert to ask permission to come and do rituals to his ancestors on the farm. Little did we know that he was establishing a false precedent for a land claim. According to George, never before had this clan expressed any interest in their ancestors' graves. When the claim finally surfaced, I became incensed when he called one day because I knew that, according to the principles of the Restitution Act, there was no legal claim. On the phone he threatened me, and on a separate occasion George as well, saying that he had powerful medicine that could kill George if he continued to support me.

Concerning the dark forces, never offer a challenge!
Never be disrespectful of the dark forces, neither underestimate
their power nor over-estimate your own dealing with them.
Avoidance, when possible, is best.

It became clear that Silas was going to be working against us, not only through the legal system, which he seemed to have mastered, but also with witchcraft, to ensure the claim would be successful. Later on we realized he was also coming to work his witchcraft locally on the land. Although we were somewhat reluctant to allow him to come and do rituals, we could not legally prevent him from coming onto the farm to visit the graves as long as he asked permission, and that he was always careful to do.

We would lay down our own protective medicine to counteract his witchcraft and that of his witch associates, and with the help of Andries both George and I became quite expert in repelling their negative intentions. This was a constant battle, requiring us to renew the defenses from time to time. Whenever I would be leaving to go back to the United States, I would always go with George and visit Andries to make sure that he was amply protected during my absence. Andries was reassuring that we were well-guarded by the ancestors and by his methods, and that as long as we were attentive we should not really worry too much about it.

What impressed me most about Andries were not only his profound *sangoma* abilities, but also his spiritual integrity, and especially his attitude towards witchcraft. He never attempted to counter it by bewitching the perpetrator, in this case Silas. His method was rather to defend and block it as opposed to using negative power himself. He explained that a *sangoma* who works in the light never aligns with dark forces to curse a witch, but rather, like a mirror, reflects the evil intention back to the one who sent it. His approach was entirely in line with what we had been taught by the ancestors. Andries seemed aware that using witchcraft himself would have serious karmic implications.

Good prevails by being what it is, not by dispossessing, defeating or winning, but rather simply by being more and more of what it is.

Nevertheless, there were a few disturbing threats. The first was when I was nearly thrown out of my bed by "tilo." The second was an incident that occurred just before a group was due to arrive from the United States.

I was getting things ready for the visit. Before any group came, George would always check on the trails and make sure that the head-high grass was not too long, so that everyone could walk in the bush with less fear of ticks and snakes. Daily hikes, especially with the focus on *muti*, were a big part of the *sangoma* experience. The large baobab tree on the property was particularly beautiful, with huge rocky outcrops around it. I asked George to cut a trail to the tree so that the group could walk there safely and go and sit on the rocks to meditate. Strangely, I had never asked him to do this before for any of the other groups. George went down with Simon, and both were cutting the long grass on the approach to the baobab. As they approached the tree, George got a sickening feeling and looked in the tree. A triangular slot had been cut out, in which he saw a pot, the mouth of which appeared to be pointing at the *Tshisimane* homestead above. George came up the hill to relay his concern that there was serious witchcraft afoot. We drove back down to the tree and sure enough, in the baobab trunk, a triangular slot had been carved out where rituals of some sort must have been offered in times past, possibly even negative ones against Bos, the missionary. The baobab is unusual in that it can reline its own bark and can even survive the ring-barking that may occur when browsing elephants strip a tree. This triangle in the tree had been intentionally cut, and was just big enough to accommodate a quite beautiful ceramic pot that seemed to be pointing towards the house, almost like a satellite dish. It felt ominous. The triangle had been relined with bark, indicating that it had been cut many years previously and used before. George suggested we go down to Andries and consult with him.

When we arrived at Andries', George described the circumstances concerning the pot. I was surprised when Andries turned to me and said, "This is a snake!" To me it looked like a pot, but Andries, being well versed in the ancient laws of the malevolent occult, thought otherwise. Venda witches and sorcerers have been plying their dark skills expertly for eons, and Andries had considerable experience in counteracting such situations. I could not understand what he was telling me, but I believed him.

Andries seemed very concerned, and he and his three *sangoma* wives jumped into the pickup and we drove them back to the farm. When we arrived at the baobab, Andries took out a genet-skin bag in which he kept some black protective medicine. He carefully took the pot out of the tree and smeared the whole thing with the *muti*, then hit it with the bag. He took the pot, aimed it at the triangular slot in the tree, and threw it. The pot not only went precisely inside the nook in the tree, but shattered completely, with all the malevolent contents of the pot and the shards remaining inside the tree. Needless to say, none of us wanted to look further as to what may have been the contents. Andries wiped his hands on the ground and said, "It's finished. You do not need to worry. You are safe now. You can take us home." You could see by the expression on all of their faces that they had been very worried about what could have happened.

I returned to the house to ponder the pot that was a snake but that wasn't. The group from the USA arrived the next day and as I was making some introductory remarks to them in the healing hut, I looked up and saw George's worried face at the door of the hut. He said, "Dave, you need to come and look." I walked with him and the group followed me. Some ten yards from the kitchen door of the house was a five-foot mfesi, or Mozambique spitting cobra, that George had just killed. George and I looked at each other and we silently acknowledged Andries' wisdom and the steps he had taken to protect us. I later came to understand that the pot had been a "container" to send the snake to bite one of us, especially at the time when the group was going to be there and there was a greater possibility for collateral damage. If it had not been for George finding the pot, and Andries' timely intervention, the story could have ended tragically, more especially so if one of the group had been bitten.

A second incident happened with a later group when a smaller mfesi reared up on someone doing a meditation walk in the labyrinth. She was not bitten, but dislocated one finger in her hand as she tripped and fell while trying to back away. It was significant that there had been a group of nine people who had signed on for that particular trip. Prior to the date of the trip, I received messages from my ancestors that the "dark forces" were congregating and collaborating in creating havoc with this particular group, two of whom were respected and powerful healers. After checking with the bones, I ended up taking only three of the nine who had applied to come, and the two healers were excluded. One was particularly upset because she felt that her guides were powerful enough to protect us all. The other healer at first was disappointed, but checked in with her guides and after that was relieved to not be going. She said that she saw a dark cloud looming over the trip that looked ominous. Fortunately all turned out well with the woman and her damaged hand, but it may have been different if there were too many "variables" to control. Tricksters, dark forces and witches love to cause trouble, especially when the stakes are high and there is more potential for doing harm or for undermining the credibility of their opposition. There were never any other snake incidents in all the years I spent at *Tshisimane*, in spite of the prevalence of mambas and mfesi.

Witches use familiars on which they can "travel," and which can be energetically manipulated to ambush a person on their path. Familiars other than snakes include baboons, genets, wild cats, owls and hyenas. We had frequently experienced owls hooting or brown hyenas prowling at night when witchcraft was afoot.

It should be noted that although this chapter is about witchcraft, that for those on a shamanic or any spiritual journey, there are also independent dark forces on the other side of the veil that will try to thwart their higher purpose. The deeper one's commitment to working in the light, the sooner one becomes visible to these trickster spirits. Negative entities will try, by any means possible, to sabotage one's progress. The more connected a witch or sorcerer is to these entities, the more powerful he or she is, but it is important to realize that the same dark forces can work entirely independently from witchcraft and on their own behalf.

> *The contest between light and dark is most fierce when the stakes are high. We may expect to be challenged, tempted and dissuaded in any and all manner of our weaknesses, be they physical, mental or emotional, all of which are attributes of the spirit.*

This is sometimes called a "costly compliment."

When I relate these stories to skeptics and sense their disbelief, I remember that a few years previously I also may not have credited these explanations. My attitude, after several years at *Tshisimane*, changed radically.

There is a particular medicinal plant, now almost extinct but legendary in Limpopo and beyond, that can be used for good or for bad, depending on one's intention, and of course, Silas' intention was not one of doing good. He had said to George once, "If you go, Dave will go," and he knew that my weak underbelly was my total reliance on George. George handled the property when I was gone and I depended on him to take care of everything. We suspected that Silas had managed to procure some of this medicine for his use, and he had even boasted about it on at least one occasion.

Andries had divined that Silas was working with three very experienced witches in the village, but that with the methods he gave us, we would be able to counteract their attacks. This relentless fight to stave off these challenges became quite tedious and exhausting over the years. We managed to defend and prevail against the malevolence, at least on a day-to-day basis, but at times it became difficult to follow the ancestors' directive ...

Think of something that makes your heart glad that can bring you back to equanimity. The dark forces are most helpless in the face of love and laughter.

Other times we felt much lighter, such as when George told me that Silas was now frightened to come onto the property, and even though he would call to say he wanted to visit, he would not show up on the appointed day. George was getting the message from the village down below that Silas was becoming scared of us because all the things that he had tried to do had not really worked, and in some instances may have backfired. George related a story that he had heard of Silas going to see a new witch who had declined to help him because he said we seemed to be fairly impermeable to the most expert spells. Silas also once bragged to his friends in the village that I would not be coming to *Tshisimane* anymore because of the effectiveness of his work. Shortly afterward I arrived in my red *bakkie* and he lost face. Nevertheless, we took nothing for granted and assumed that the attacks would continue unless we finally packed up and left *Tshisimane.*

I met Rupert shortly before the turn of the millennium. We became good friends, but at that time were clearly miles apart in terms of our belief systems. He often said to me, "Dave, I know there is another realm out there, but I am really not sure about a lot of the stuff that you talk about."

When I first met him we went on a hike down a beautiful river, and even though it was exquisite with pools and subtropical forest, I did not like the energy in some of the places. When we were walking down the river we sat down for a rest and Rupert said, "It's a shame that we do not have time to go to one of the pools that is further on, because it's amazing, and there is an interesting cave there I would like you to see."

He told me how on one occasion he had gone into the cave and seen three beautiful ceramic pots. He had also noticed that there were puff adder skins around them, with the heads of the deadly snakes perched on top in a formidable protective fashion. This had not daunted Rupert, who had removed the skins and taken the pots home. When I first heard this story, I said, "Rupert, you have to be out of your mind! You need to take those pots back!" Rupert did not understand my concern at the time and declined to do so.

Rupert was a gifted jazz musician and an excellent tour guide, but he did not seem to be getting the work he deserved. He told me how, initially, he had played the trumpet, but one day had fallen off his bicycle, smashing his jaw. After that he could no longer play. Hence he was playing keyboard when we first met. I also noted that the little finger of one hand was not straight because of a ruptured tendon that had subsequently occurred. This forced him to play the keyboard with only nine fingers. These events both postdated the ceramic pot heist.

When I came back on a subsequent visit, he told me how he had ruptured his biceps tendon in one arm and had been out of work for two months in a cast. Then a year later when I arrived he was again in a cast, having just ruptured the biceps tendon of the other arm, and again could not play for another two months. It was at this stage that Rupert came to me and said, "Dave, maybe you need to throw the bones. It seems like something is trying to attack me and it always has something to do with my music and my ability to make a living." Apart from these events, Rupert was a healthy, powerful, fit man who should have had no issues with his tendons.

I threw the bones, but actually I knew what they were going to say. They confirmed the fact that his house was bewitched. I told Rupert that he had to take the pots back to the cave, make an offering, and give an apology for what he had done. I gave him medicines to protect his house, as well as to protect him along the way. He did finally go back and do all the necessary things, and since that time his life and luck have turned around. Rupert has become a firm believer in the *sangoma* paradigm and frequently requests divinations.

Concerning the dark forces: Purity of intent and impeccability is your greatest defense. Actually no defense is needed in the face of total surrender to the Divine despite the intensity of the attack, temptation or persuasiveness. If commitment to the light is total then the dark forces cannot prevail. The challenge is to dedicate yourself to this no matter how it feels. Determination and steadfastness of will withstand even the darkest force with equanimity and even merriment. If you would dispel the darkness, fill the space with light.

XVII

Land claims

You cannot control results, only your actions. You cannot decide outcomes, only your choices.

God does not measure results but only the trueness of intent and the fervor of effort. This is why there is such joy in daring one's best for love of God.

WHEN SOUTH AFRICA GAINED INDEPENDENCE FOR THE first time and Mandela came into power, both he and Bishop Tutu decided that there had to be land restitution. The intention was to restore land that had been confiscated from blacks by the apartheid government and placed in white hands. The Restitution Act that was introduced was a just act and the parameters were laid out very clearly. There was a statute of limitations so that claims were not valid for land residing in the hands of whites before apartheid was formally instituted. To have a valid claim, the claimants had to prove that they had ancestral graves on the land and that the apartheid government had forcefully evicted them. The hope was to restore at least 30% of white-owned property back to the original black families.

Unfortunately, the principles of the Restitution Act became corrupted, and eventually land claims resulted in a free-for-all in which the basic parameters were ignored by the authorities. There was a cutoff date for land claims, but claims continued to surface long after the cutoff date. There were even stories of foreign residents who lodged totally illegal claims. Almost anyone could claim that they had ancestral graves, especially on particularly desirable pieces of real estate. Today the government admits that the policy was a failure, and the Land Claims program is defunct as of this writing.

When I first bought Uniondale in 2002, land claims were the furthest thing from my mind, although I was aware of the fact that they were becoming an issue. As of 2002 no land claim had surfaced on the farm, so I felt reassured. After I took up residence and started to build, the land claim surfaced. I thought it was spurious and would be rejected, but it was not long before it was officially gazetted and became real. Silas, who instigated the claim, had already been coming to the farm intermittently to do rituals to his ancestors. I realized, in retrospect, that he had been laying the groundwork for a land claim. He wanted validation for the fact that there were ancestral graves on the land that he said belonged to his clan. Since I had felt guided there by the ancestors and knew the claim to be illegal, I did not take it all too seriously in the beginning, mistakenly thinking that I would prevail in court if a claim were lodged. Certainly there were graves, and so I decided to start learning about the history of *Tshisimane*.

It was in the early stages of Uniondale becoming *Tshisimane* that I had the dream to buy Calitzdorp. I had no need for another 700 hectares of land but the dream, which occurred twice in one night, was so compelling that I purchased it. I could not understand why the ancestors were so insistent, but believed it was necessary for some reason or other that would become

clear. Shortly after I bought Calitzdorp land claims surfaced
there as well, in spite of guarantees by my attorney that none
existed when I bought it. I now thought that Calitzdorp might
be a bargaining factor in my being able to keep *Tshisimane*,
where all the development had been done. Claimants had the
option of keeping the land if the claim was validated or, if
they preferred, being paid compensation by the government. I
hoped that if it came to that they would keep Calitzdorp and
be happy to be paid out for Uniondale/ *Tshisimane*.

I received notification that one of the Land Claim commis-
sioners would be coming out with the clan to inspect the land
and visit the graves, notably the "chief's" grave. The whole clan
arrived with Silas, in a series of pickups. We all marched off
to visit the grave with the commissioner. It was under a huge
rocky edifice in a very pristine area on Calitzdorp. The commissioner turned around to me and said, "You are, of course,
going to acknowledge this claim, aren't you?" I replied, "If it is a
valid claim I would be happy to do so, but from what I can see
the claim is not legal." My comment did not receive a warm reception. There were several old ladies present who argued that
they had been there at the time the police had come, beaten
them, thrown them into trucks and taken them away. I knew
this was not true since George was born on the property and
his grandfather and father had worked there. Both George's
grandfather and father were also buried on Calitzdorp, and if
anyone had a claim, he did. He knew the whole history of the
area, and the farmers who had been there had never mistreated
the Venda people who had lived and worked on Uniondale
and Calitzdorp. Neither had there been any evictions by the
apartheid regime. The Dutch missionary, Bos, had bought the
upper farm, Uniondale, in 1898, and it was abundantly clear

that both of these farms had been in white hands long before the date for a claim to become legal. The commissioner, who was clearly biased, seemed unconcerned with these details and fully supported the claim. Bos had started a school and the headman, whose grave we were attending, had died of old age. He had been buried at the foot of a rocky outcrop. I had never before visited the area because it was sequestered in some thick bush. This proved to be a grave mistake.

When we arrived at what George told me had originally been a few stones that marked the grave, we were greeted with a semblance of a small cemetery. Silas had been building his case for a claim while we trusted he had just been making offerings to the ancestors. The headman's now elongated grave had an impressive mound of stones on top of it, and there were more small circular stone demarcations where Silas assured us that the chief's wives had been buried in the traditional way, sitting upright. It was a mystery to me why the headman would not have been buried this way as well, but probably Silas realized a longitudinal grave with a large mound would be more impressive and "chief-like." George later told me that no wives had been buried there whatsoever, and that Silas had advanced the idea that the headman was actually a "chief" to empower the claim. Silas also proclaimed himself son of the chief, which was only partially true. He was the illegitimate child of one of the headman's consorts. He had become his own pretender to a fictitious title of Chief and was already acting like one to the rest of the clan. He even charged them fees to cover his "expenses" when he had claim meetings with them.

George and others had told me that gradually, as work developed in the cities, people had migrated away from the farms to seek more lucrative employment. No one had been forcefully evicted from either of these farms, an essential prerequisite to a valid claim. At the time I was incensed by the injustice of it all, but this was to change as I slowly researched my various options in the face of the stark realities of the prevailing system.

Now I was in the situation of having both farms under claim. It was up to me to prove that the claims were invalid. I was guilty until I proved otherwise. I knew that it was going to cost me a lot of money, not only in legal fees but also in anthropology research and possibly even aerial photographs if I was to prove my case. The claimants' costs, however, were to be covered by Land Claims. I wondered why I had been sent there by my ancestors, only to find later that the land was going to be expropriated. I was especially puzzled by the dream to also purchase Calitzdorp.

The apartheid regime had kept excellent records in Pretoria. I confirmed with others, including an anthropologist, that there had been no evictions and that the stories of the old ladies being thrown into trucks and being beaten were lies. George told me that rather than chasing anyone off the land, some of the farmers had urged those who had left for the cities to return. It was clear to me that none of this would make any difference in court. George was prepared to testify on my behalf, but I was not going to run the risk of having him harmed or even killed for it on my account.

At this stage Calitzdorp had been cleaned up and the building at *Tshisimane* was complete. Rupert said to me, "I am sure that if you would not have done all this work, there would never have been a land claim." There had been no interest in the farms until I came and began developing them. Rupert was even more incensed than I was and called the whole debacle sheer piracy.

I went about my research in a systematic fashion. I first

consulted an anthropologist, who was supposed to come out to the farm on numerous occasions but never showed up. It became apparent that he was much more interested in the larger, more lucrative farms in the area than he was in my humble property. Many of these were farms or wilderness retreats and tourist attractions. Fortunately he assigned me another anthropologist whom I really liked and who proved to be a tremendous asset. He had access to all the pertinent records through Pretoria's archives. He researched the issue for a very reasonable cost. At the end of the day he came back to me and said, "Dave, there were no evictions, and there is no valid claim on the land, but you will lose anyway. Give it up!" This was sobering advice from somebody who obviously would gain more money if he were to have to come to court and testify on my behalf. He stood in contrast to some anthropologists who were doing exceedingly well financially by telling the farmers that all would be well if they continued the fight.

I also researched the subject with some prominent lawyers in Johannesburg who dealt exclusively with land claims. Here I got a taste of reality from one who said, "The probability of you winning a land claim in court is most unlikely." They recommended that I relinquish the claim and work out an agreement with the family to lease it back from them after they took it over. This option left a sour taste in my mouth because Silas would no doubt exploit his position of power, and I did not care to rent or have anything to do with anyone that unsavory.

I had already had a meeting with the family some time before this visit. I had hoped that I could keep Uniondale/*Tshisimane* while they could have the more commercially viable Calitzdorp. They would then be compensated for Uniondale. I was told that this was not negotiable and that they wanted both parcels.

They said I should maintain and rent their land from them as a compromise. The Restitution Act stated that if the claim was valid, the claimants could take over the property, while the owner, usually white, would be paid out with the fair market value. The claimants, however, had to show that they had expertise to manage the land, or farm, or business. In my case there was no expertise required to manage the properties. However, in many other instances there were sophisticated farms, game lodges or wilderness retreats for which suitable training was required. In these cases Land Claims would appoint a manager, who would assist the claimants until such time as they could take it over themselves. All of this, although logical, did not turn out to be very effective in the long run, and many of the farms that were taken over were soon in disrepair.

There was a remote possibility that the landowner might prevail in the claim and that the claim would be dismissed, but I knew of no such instance taking place. The best option usually favored both by Land Claims and the claimants was to relinquish the land and work out an agreement with the claimants to lease or rent back from them. In other words, "pay to stay." This was not an option for me in lieu of the negative cash flow I was already experiencing, and more especially because of Silas, who was less trustworthy than the mambas who continued to warn me about him in and out of my dreams.

I also consulted with a few of the local farmers who were being subjected to land claims, especially those in the rich agricultural area of Luvubu. They advised me to get out as soon as possible, since the first ones in the areas to submit were usually the ones who were given the best prices. They said there was a tendency for prices to diminish after the first few farmers surrendered their land. I was also told that once the farms were claimed, property values fell, because many of the farms deteriorated after being transferred. This was in spite of managers being appointed where necessary. Farming is competitive and requires a lot of hard work, dedication and sophisticated knowledge. Even if an expert manager was appointed, it is unlikely he would put the same passion into the land as a farmer whose family had lived there for generations. It also was unlikely that somebody who had just inherited a farm, without really having to work for it, would have enough passion to make a success of it. There were instances in which farmers had rented their farms back from the claimants and continued to farm successfully. There were even some others where the farmer had relinquished his land and then bought it back at a later date at a much lower price and then continued to farm.

A friend of mine in Port Elizabeth, who did environmental impact reviews for many of the farms in her area and was very well informed, advised me to relinquish the claim and possibly think of leasing it back. This overall had proven the most successful strategy.

Around that time I had several dreams that were very disturbing. In one dream an aunt of mine appeared and asked, "Are you prepared to die for this place?" I had been feeling that even if I won the claim I would in effect lose, because there would still be ongoing witchcraft, not to mention pilfering and poaching, especially when I was away. This was already happening on other farms and there had even been several farm murders in the area. In another dream a voice said to me, "You should buy a gun when you go back." In a third dream I was told that I should learn the Israeli special forces form of self-defense called *Kav Magar*. I did not want to feel that I was in a war or witchcraft zone in order to hang on to the land, no matter how compelling and magical it was.

The most seminal dream was as follows: I was being towed through the water by a speedboat, and I was holding onto a chain for dear life. I managed to inch my way up the chain towards the boat to avoid drowning, and eventually was able to climb into the boat. The boat then docked and the fellow docking it said to me, "You made it out just in time."

Based on this, I decided to "pull out in time and avoid drowning." This tied in with similar advice I had from a *sangoma* friend, as well as from someone who worked high up in government circles. The *sangoma* told me that if I were to surf the chat rooms on the web, I would find that there was a lot of sympathy in South Africa for the way Mugabe had handled land issues. He had just expropriated farms from the whites in Zimbabwe, often violently. All of this was also influenced by the fact that I had a perfectly good life in California.

It became clear that it was time to go. As a lesson in non-attachment it was also good spiritual practice. I started to regard *Tshisimane* much in the way that a Tibetan Buddhist would regard one of their painstakingly made, beautiful sand-painted mandalas. After spending many months making one, they would destroy it to show their commitment to the concept of impermanence, the importance of surrender, and the simple but profound spiritual principle of being in the present moment. If someone were to ask, which some did, "Why ever did you surrender?" I would defer to the ancestors ...

Surrender fortifies, not weakens. It does not diminish
desire nor dilute determination. It is the eyes of trust
that see what seeing eyes do not. Surrender is a giving in.
Resignation is a giving up!

To me, surrender meant letting go and not holding on to some ideal that no longer existed except in the past. Resignation meant being attached to the past in spite of overwhelming odds against a happy outcome, whether I won (most unlikely) or lost. Even if I won the battle, there was no doubt I would lose the war.

When I looked back at my stay at *Tshisimane*, I decided that I had already realized most of the benefits that could have accrued. There would be steadily diminishing returns after this. I had significantly deepened my knowledge of *sangoma* medicine, especially with reference to the medicinal plants in the area and how they worked. For this reason alone, I felt that I had achieved what I wanted to do. I became more philosophical than angry, and the previous dream messages reassured me that I did not need a healing center. My job was to "take from there to bring to here" (the USA), not the other way around. There are 250,000 *sangomas* in South Africa – the country would manage without one more. The only confusing factor to me now was, why the dream to purchase Calitzdorp? The reason for this was to become clear.

I told Land Claims that I would agree to the claim, and we worked towards that. Following this, and even before, my relationships with all those concerned with the claim in the Polokwane office – except for the one commissioner who had visited the farm, who later was dismissed – were highly professional and commendable. A land claim assessor came to evaluate the property, and George showed him around in my absence. The assessment went according to square footage, and a certain amount of money was assigned to each area accordingly. It did not really matter how good the quality of the building was, which was lucky for me since *Tshisimane* was extremely rustic.

There had been no significant financial outlay on Calitzdorp, and most of the money had gone into building *Tshisimane*. I expected to get a decent return on *Tshisimane*, and because there was not much development at Calitzdorp, I was less optimistic about that. However, *Tshisimane* was only an aesthetically pleasing property perched on top of a mountain – extremely beautiful, but without commercial value. It could not really be farmed and, because of the thick bush and mountainous terrain, was not suitable for cattle. This was not the case with Calitzdorp, which had plentiful water, excellent farmland, and good cattle grazing. In fact there were cattle on it from the time that I bought the property. These usually belonged to members of George's family, who had nowhere else to allow their cattle to graze.

The one problem with cattle was that there was a huge tick infestation around the homestead. This made it intolerable for Silas when he came back once to look over the property. I never received any payment for allowing the cattle to graze, and was occasionally bothered by the ticks when I would visit. When I heard from George about the torment they caused Silas on his visit, I admit to being glad about the cattle and the tick bonanza's effects on Silas. Tiny, almost invisible, pepper ticks can burrow under the skin, usually settling in the groin area, where they can create severe itching for weeks.

It took several months for the assessment to be completed. When I returned to *Tshisimane*, I went to meet the Land Claims officials in Makhado to hear how they had evaluated the farm. The appraisal proved the reverse of what I had anticipated. Calitzdorp was commercially more valuable than Uniondale, in spite of the money invested in the latter. It then became apparent to me why I had been instructed by the ancestors to buy Calitzdorp. I had bought both Uniondale and Calitzdorp for R1000 per hectare. I received the same for Uniondale, in spite of the buildings and all the development in creating *Tshisimane*. However, for Calitzdorp I received R1600 per hectare. This made up for my losses at Uniondale. At the end of the day I came out more or less even, except for all the work and for the loss of income due to time spent away from my medical practice and travel back and forth from California.

Since then I am always reluctant to try to second-guess advice coming to me from the other side of the veil between worlds. I felt a tremendous sense of gratitude for the dream that made me buy the Calitzdorp farm I had never wanted. Though I was advised that the price I was given was fair, for peace of mind I had a second assessment done by an independent assessor. He concurred with the price, and I accepted it.

By now I had already noticed a change of mood in the area. There seemed to be a sense of gloom amongst many of my farmer friends. Almost every farm on that part of the mountain had been claimed, regardless of whether there was a valid claim or not. Hendrik's farm at the bottom of the mountain along the Sand River had also been claimed, and the minute this happened he became even more bad-tempered than before. His ire was not particularly directed towards me, but towards his own land. He seemed to lose respect for it, and made a contract with a mining company to come and mine the sand in the Sand River that fronted his property. Bulldozers, backhoes, trucks and noise now marred the previously tranquil and scenic drive up to *Tshisimane*, and he intensified his hunting. I felt even more reconciled to it that I would be leaving this mess behind. The sand mining was undercutting the access dirt road that skirted that part of the river, and there was concern that if there was a significant rain the river might wash it away. This had already happened during the major floods in 2000. It made me even more reconciled about my decision to leave.

The ancestors' dream wisdom and advice made it much easier for me to leave my wilderness sanctuary. I was paid out in full just barely before the Land Claims office declared bankruptcy. Knowing my guides had a hand in the happy closure, I am profoundly grateful to them. The ancestors previously had advised that I should be prepared to walk away without any settlement at all. I had hoped and prayed otherwise, and could not have anticipated a better outcome. I also realized that the land claims and the successful settlement were freeing me from being tied down to *Tshisimane* long-term, which might have proved crippling to my destiny path. I was only meant to be there for that brief but fruitful period. I had fulfilled my dream.

Hope is about believing, in spite of the evidence, and then watching the evidence change.

Trust your affairs to the Lord and your plans will succeed. To know this is wisdom, to act on this is faith.

Be grateful and you will be happy. Happiness leads to great empowerment. Attend to your well being, especially to happiness, the cause for which is sometimes found in hidden recesses, always in gratitude.

XVIII

The End

Stay close to the ancestors' guidance.

I WAS NOW FACED WITH THE TASK OF FREEING MYSELF FROM all the investments in *Tshisimane*. This included the setting up of a whole homestead, a home away from home. I reconciled myself that it was not about the destination but about the journey, and this had been valuable, meaningful and magical in more ways than I could describe.

The furnishings in *Tshisimane* and how they had been set up were a whole other story. Most had been brought up the road with a 4x4 and a trailer. The cupboards and beds could not be transported up the challenging track and were built at *Tshisimane*. They were made out of heavy eucalyptus and, although very rustic, fitted the ambience well. My new work now consisted of dismantling the entire *Tshisimane* dream and trying to ensure that when Silas took it over it would be entirely empty of all the "non-fixed" assets.

The ancestors again seemed to be on my side, and what seemed like a daunting task proceeded without any difficulty. I took the tractor and trailer back to Luvubu to Henry and left it there to sell. Some months later he sold them both for a reasonable price. They had been indispensable in the building of *Tshisimane* and had been trouble free.

This was my first successful exit coup. The next thing was to get rid of all the furnishings, solar, wind and gasoline generators, batteries, stove and fridge, to mention only the basics. I spoke to an auctioneer, who laughed and said nobody would come up that road and, even if they would, how would they bring the stuff down? He told me to give it away or just let it go, maybe even leave it for the claimants.

I called Leon Oosthuizen, who had sold me the property. Leon had a magnificent farm higher up on the mountain and loved to have extra things on hand, which he always needed. When I told him that I was leaving, he agreed to take everything off my hands for 50% of the cost price. In a series of trips, Leon came with his truck and some workers and took just about everything, leaving *Tshisimane* relatively empty. The only things of value left behind were the water pump and water heaters, that were fixtures and had to remain.

We were now left with the bare essentials: a two-burner gas stove, a small gas fridge, and hurricane kerosene lanterns. *Tshisimane* felt much like it had when I first arrived. I enjoyed going back to this simplicity, but there was a certain lonely emptiness now about the place. I gave George the pickup, the appliances and the gas containers that serviced the hot water heaters, as well as all the tools, chain saws, etc. in the workshop. I was gratified that *Tshisimane* would be totally empty by the time George left.

I had previously been trying to get George work in some of the surrounding areas, but to no avail. Shortly before I left, I received a call from Ian at Lajuma. Ian ran an educational center where he accepted university students from abroad, most of whom were studying zoology. He had some fascinating projects on his farm, especially the research he was doing on leopards. I had approached him previously about employing George, but at that time he had had no need for him. Now Ian said he would take George on.

There had been some issue as to whether George would choose to stay on at the Calitzdorp farm. According to the Restitution Act, he was fully entitled to remain. In fact George was more entitled than anyone else, but he was the only one who had not joined the claimants.

I had a long talk with George and said to him, "You know that once I leave, if you stay, the opposition to you and the witchcraft will not stop. They do not like you any more than they like me, and they will give you no peace. You will constantly have to be on the defensive and watching your back. Maybe this isn't worthwhile."

Although George felt he could not trust Silas, he decided to go down the mountain and make his peace with him and the rest of the claimants. He was hopeful that now that they had prevailed and I was leaving, something might change. Unlike Silas, the clan in general had not been too adversarial toward George or myself during the claim.

However, they certainly resented him for being faithful to his white employer. George told me that when he chatted with the family Silas' mother said in Afrikaans, "*Hy word moeg,*" meaning he is getting tired—he is done with fighting—he is giving up. Silas, always sly like a fox, was very friendly and said to him, "Now that Dave is gone, everything will be different, and you can stay on." George believed him, knowing that this was in line with the law and the concept of restitution, which stipulated that all those who had ancestral graves and were connected to the claim were entitled. Silas told him he could live in the Calitzdorp house. George thought that this gesture was possibly because of the tick infestation. George went ahead and upgraded the small house at Calitzdorp. He burned the surrounding grass to reduce the ticks and planted maize and spinach. He hoped that now, due to the reconciliation with Silas, he might remain there peacefully. His intention was to practice as a *sangoma* there since Calitzdorp, being at the bottom of the mountain, was quite accessible from the village. George also hoped that once the claim was finalized, the family would be smart enough to take control away from Silas. This was not to happen, however; they all appeared to be too afraid of Silas and his witchcraft antics.

The day I was about to leave *Tshisimane* for the last time, Hendrik, my problematic neighbor, finally received what was due to him. George was driving up the hill in his newly-acquired *bakkie* just as I was ready to drive out in my rental. George came into the empty house with a big smile on his face and told me the story.

He said he had been driving up past the Sand River only to find Hendrik coming down in his pickup. A truck full of sand was coming out of the river. Hendrik jumped out of his pickup, ran up to the truck and accosted the black driver. Hendrik had been a policeman in the apartheid days, but apartheid was now dead. Hendrik was furious and had also forgotten his manners. He grabbed the driver by the shirt and started to scream and curse at him in Afrikaans, saying that he had not been paid for his sand. This man, however, had no control over the finances, he just drove the truck. The driver got out of the truck and knocked Hendrik to the ground and began to kick him. George laughed even more when he told me this part of the story since he said that the driver of the vehicle was much smaller than Hendrik and even walked with a limp. A piece of lead pipe was lying in the sand, and the driver stooped to pick it up. Hendrik saw what was about to happen, cowered and screamed even louder, now in terror of having his head bashed in. George, who was watching, shouted to the driver; "No, don't do it, you will get into big trouble, it's not worth it." The driver backed off while Hendrik ran back to his pickup, screaming that he was going to go and get his gun and shoot him and anyone else around. When I drove down the mountain and past Hendrik's house I had a big smile on my face. Hendrik was nowhere in sight.

Epilogue

When Silas eventually took possession of the two farms, he gave George three hours to remove all of his stuff and to get out of Calitzdorp. This required that George rent a truck to haul his belongings away. Silas would not even allow him to come and pick the crop he had planted. All along he had schemed to benefit from George's work and investments in the house.

George completed his initiation as a *sangoma* and continued to have guidance and dreams from his grandfather. It was a strange reversal that the reason he became a *sangoma* was because of a white person. It had never been a consideration for him until we became friends.

Silas continued with his devious plots and was cited by the authorities for cutting down trees in the nature conservancy that is now a biosphere. For a short while a church made a deal with him and took over *Tshisimane* in exchange for giving him a secondhand *bakkie*. They were holding services there, but the road must have defied them and they did not remain. George had only been back once to help the claimants sort out the complicated water system, but the pump has since seized up and the well is useless. The claimants removed all the protective wire on the thatch roof to use or sell, and the baboons have ripped the thatch apart. They have taken over the homestead, as they also did at Calitzdorp, and nature has reclaimed *Tshisimane*. The neighbors at the top of the mountain say that the road is in disrepair and full of trash that accumulates again immediately after they pick it up. In George's words, *Tshisimane "hy is kla"* – it's finished! Silas' *bakkie* is no more, he is in ever decreasing health, and he is more impoverished than ever. The last I heard was that he had left the village and was running away from the police after a murder. Again the ancestors are proved correct …

"What you destroy, destroys you. What you defeat, defeats you. What you sanctify, sanctifies you."

Silas, in spite of winning the claim, had done nothing to sanctify his life or that of the witches who worked on his behalf, all of whom I understood from George were either sick or had passed on.

I used to go back and renew my connection with George on a yearly basis. We would swap stories of our *sangoma* experiences and he would renew my *muti* supplies. Sadly George passed away recently. He had always said to me that if he left the mountain and had to live in the village he would not live long. He proved himself correct. I never knew his age but assumed I was a good twenty years older than him. I remember him fondly and the challenges we faced together.

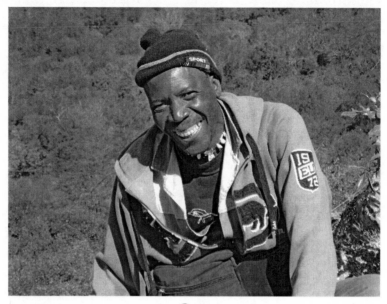

George

I am grateful to have had the opportunity to live out a dream and to have learned so much from the mysterious land and people of Venda. It still remains my favorite place in all of Southern Africa.

When I return to the Soutpansberg I stay with friends. I still have not had the courage to visit *Tshisimane*. The *Tshisimane* sign no longer stands on the road between Makhado and Vivo just as you cross the Sand River. When Mandela came to power after the fall of apartheid, I had fancied that I could return to my roots and, as a surgeon turned *sangoma*, make a contribution to the place of my birth. This was not to be. I return to my South African watering hole to get replenished about once a year—to walk in the bush, visit the old healers, and arrange the new dream songs with Eugene. Whenever I come back home and drive into Santa Barbara, I feel a profound gratitude for my life in California.

If the burden were taken away the lesson would not be learned. Coping with it is what is important and what counts.

Reveal always truth and you will be guided about what to do.

Since being initiated, and even more so after leaving Tshismane, I have been living in two worlds. I still have a surgical practice in Santa Barbara, California where I operate and dispense allopathic medicine. I also practice indigenous healing out of my home. There I have an *ndumba* where I divine with the bones and dispense *mutis* and rituals for the various ailments. I still prefer Western medicine for standard complaints like infections, trauma, cancer and so forth, where the bones are no substitute for a CT scan or an MRI. On the other hand, Western medicine is sadly lacking in the spiritual dimensions, and I have found the combination of the two paradigms ideal. Patients may come for this help once the complaint has been eradicated by Western technology, to find out what they can do to improve their inner balance and prevent other diseases. Others may come if Western medicine has failed them. Still others come for problems not related to their physical health. I prefer to think of the work I do in my office and the operating room as the "curing," or at least the attempt at "curing," whereas the ministering I do in the *ndumba* is the "healing." Many patients are cured by Western technology but remain unhealed, and may go on to develop other maladies. The bones will sometimes reveal a previously unrealized psycho-socio-spiritual problem that has given no symptoms. Recognizing and treating this occult imbalance can prevent the "dis-ease," and eventually the possibility of organic disease developing as well. One can be cured of disease but still not be healed, and vice versa.

Symptoms are never not present but frequently are so subtle, camouflaged and obscured that they are not discernible or recognizable. So do not overlook the unlikely because they can be hidden and undetectable. Also do not be dismissive because the symptoms may masquerade as something else. Do not too readily accept the obvious —you may need to go beyond it.

Curing is not necessary for healing, though healing may effect a cure.

APPENDIX 1

sangoma medicine and how it works

The ancients would ask you to perform good deeds, speak good words and think good thoughts in their memory. They would want you to be a repository of their instructions, teachings and their righteous and loving ways.

The ancestors need our help just as we need theirs. Forgiveness, love and gratitude are how we help them.

THIS CHAPTER ON "HOW IT WORKS" HAS BEEN ADDED AS an appendix for those wanting more information on this amazing healing paradigm. A rudimentary understanding of *sangoma* medicine also adds to the appreciation of what it was that compelled me to build an indigenous healing center in a remote region of Limpopo. In addition, after my initiation, I felt my mission compelled me to help validate ancient Southern African healing wisdom to the West.

To most Westerners, indigenous African techniques are at best puzzling and at worst smack of witchcraft. The West is replete with technological wonders. Our communication network is a marvel with the likes of smart phones, Facebook,

Twitter and the power of the Internet. Yet ancient African wisdom has a lot to teach us about communication. There is a realm of spirit, but there is also a veil that must be penetrated if we wish to communicate with this potential source of guidance. Most Westerners do not have the techniques to pierce the veil, but *sangomas* do.

Sangoma wisdom is very practical. If you have lost a cow, the *sangoma* or the *nyanga* can go into trance or throw the bones and tell you where to go and look for it. The *sangoma's* walk is also powered by directions from his ancestors in dreams, divinations and sometimes from his colleagues. Although most *sangomas* will not throw bones for themselves, another of P.H.'s great gifts to me was to teach me to do divinations for my own journey.

There are several Bantu groups in Southern Africa. The Nguni, who are the majority, consist of the Zulu, Swazi, Xhosa and Tsonga, all of whom share a similar root language. The others are the Sotho and Tswana (similar language), and the Venda. The Venda are distinct, but have similarities to the Shona tribe in Zimbabwe. The shamans of both groups are called *sangomas* or *nyanga*s. The key to their healing states is the ability to harness *Kundalini* energy, usually without the use of mind-altering plants. The Zulu call this energy *Umbilini* and the Bushmen call it Num. *Kundalini* is latent feminine power coiled at the base of the spine which when activated by various inner practices can lead to spiritual transformation.

Sangomas, especially amongst the Nguni, use drumming and dancing to help channel the ancestors directly. All tribes obtain information from the ancestors indirectly through the medium of dreams and the divining bones. Possession or spirit mediumship among the Nguni peoples is usually overt and extroverted, whereas amongst the other tribes it had previously been more often implicit rather than explicit. However, now there is much overlap among the different groups, and drumming and possession by ancestral spirits are common to all. Trance channeling or spirit mediumship, however, was traditionally more part of the Nguni custom.

The Bantu peoples of Southern Africa, and all peoples of sub-Saharan Africa, use drumming, chanting and dancing to activate this power. Africans say, "We pray by singing and dancing." The word *sangoma* comes from the Zulu ngoma that means a drum, since it is the sound of the drum that brings forth the guiding spirit. The drumming is accompanied by special songs and chants. When the spirit enters the body, the *sangoma* becomes the channel for the ancestor who has come. Sometimes a *sangoma* will speak in tongues, and often with a different accent.

"Because of the sound of my sighing has my essence cleaved unto my flesh" (Psalm 102:5) is speaking to the soul's essence lodging comfortably in the body. Sound is not just important but crucial in breaking down or chasing away resistances. Sound shatters and crumbles barriers to the mind and heart. Sound speaks to one's vibrations. One of the best ways to cleanse and clear oneself of the cloyingness of dark forces is to dispel or change the effects of their energy with sound.

Sangomas are able to manipulate the power of belief and faith, or placebo. Placebo is a crucial tool for the *sangoma*. Western doctors, however, frequently try to eliminate the placebo effect. In Western medicine, randomized, controlled, double-blinded studies are conducted to test the true pharmacological action of a drug, unimpeded by the placebo effect or the patient's belief that the drug will work. We know that the patient's "inner healer" is able to cure many maladies if there is a strong belief in the treatment being administered. This is especially true in cases of spontaneous remission from "incurable" diseases, where studies have shown that the one overriding common denominator was a powerful faith or belief, usually based on a strong religious or spiritual foundation, that all would be well.

While Western doctors are focused on eliminating the placebo effect, *sangomas* are masters at enhancing it using their powerful rituals. Placebo is enhanced with ceremonies and plant medicines. The *muti* is always prescribed with a heavy application of imagery, attention, intention, action and affirmation. These practices have also become part of a modern integrative, or holistic, approach. Indigenous healers are usually highly influential and powerful people who are able to enter the cosmic field and invoke the help of the spirits for healing. Naturally, when the ancestors are invited to help with the healing, the remedy goes beyond placebo and would be called distant or remote healing.

The true spirit healer is one who does not pretend to empower but alerts, shows, demonstrates, shares, guides and blesses. His role is to make aware, remind, refocus and to medicate with faith, holy and practical suggestion.

Sangomas are ingenious inspirers of hope and faith. The most powerful healers reassure patients with their calm, charisma, compassion, competence and confidence. In this way the ability of the inner healer to effect a cure is maximized.

Samuel Taylor Coleridge affirmed, *"He is the best physician who is the most ingenious inspirer of hope."*

Placebo's opposite, nocebo, the power of belief to hurt, harm or even kill, is a tool of witches and sorcerers and has no place in healing. Hope is a most crucial ingredient for all healing. Engendering a lack of hope, belief, faith or trust is bad medicine. Although allopathic medicine would refute ever using the nocebo response, it is nevertheless inadvertently prevalent. When an oncologist tells his patient that he has three months to live and should go and put his affairs in order, this is a form of medical hexing. The prognosis can be as frightening and as powerful as a curse and can become a self-fulfilling prophecy. Informed consent for procedures given in a rough manner in order to satisfy a doctor's litigious fear also can be harmful to the patient's confidence in his own inner healer's ability to effect a favorable outcome.

When I was a medical student, before the days of modern imaging technology, diagnostic exploratory surgery would often be performed for cancer when the stage or even the diagnosis was in question. If the cancer was seen to be inoperable, the abdomen would be closed without anything definitive being done. For many patients this "no hope" edict was as good as a death sentence, and the patient would often perish in hospital. This was in spite of the fact that they had appeared visibly healthy on admission and now had only undergone a relatively minor exploratory procedure. The absence of any hope can immobilize the inner healer and the body's defense system and have drastic consequences.

This is reminiscent of reports from long ago when the Dutch first arrived at the Cape of Good Hope and began to colonize South Africa. When a Bushman was caught hunting and butchering domestic stock, which the Bushmen regarded as fair game, they were usually incarcerated. The jailers were often dismayed to find these healthy young men dead in their cells only a few days after being apprehended. A Bushman lives so much in the present moment he would have been incapable of understanding that there could be any hope of release from this place, so hellishly remote from his wilderness home. He would then literally "check out" because of despair.

As healers and doctors we have to be very aware of the power of nocebo and how devastating it can be, especially to those that are more vulnerable. This can be particularly so in specific instances as well as in some cultures where even today the word cancer is heard and received as a death sentence. For others the Internet can become a nocebo experience and I advise my patients to stay away from it. I will usually resist giving prognoses. I tell my patients that they are not a statistic and only the Great Spirit really knows what will happen. It would be arrogant for me to assume that I do.

As we know from reports of spontaneous remission from so-called incurable disease, the inner healer is capable of reversing almost any illness, or at least staying in balance with it. This is most likely to occur when there is an absolute belief by the patient that all will be well. Hence spontaneous remissions of advanced diseases that have defied the best that Western medicine has to offer are often more prevalent in those that are uninformed, less sophisticated, gullible, or easily convinced.

The healing of a wound must ultimately come from
the blood of the wound itself but how it is staunched,
cleansed and comforted is the healer's role. How one is
helped to one's own healing, shown and directed to its

the source

source is the ultimate role of the shaman. Any who do
otherwise are dangerously misleading if not fraudulent.

In Nguni (Zulu, Swazi, Xhosa and Tsonga) tradition, in
addition to ancestral and foreign, non-blood-root spirits, there
are terrestrial spirits, cosmic spirits and water spirits who are
very powerful. Intruder or trickster spirits may cause mischief
or get in the way of the energy flow of the living. Malicious
spirits may also be present. Malevolent entities can be exorcised by rituals or by *Femba*, a form of psychic diagnosis and
psycho-spiritual surgery or exorcism. Dark spirits are capable
of causing harm.

The *sangoma* is able to communicate with the cosmic, the
terrestrial, and the water spirits as well as with the ancestors.
The ancestors are not gods. All tribes believe in a single Great
Spirit or God (*Umkulunkulu* in Zulu, *Modimo* in Sotho), who,
however, is seen as remote and inaccessible. The ancestral spirits are there to mediate between the living and the Creator.

Since ancestral spirits may reincarnate into the same family, it is crucial to heal the wrongs that may have occurred in
the past. By reaching out, forgiving, and healing the spirit who
perpetrated any nefarious deed, everyone is healed, and a cycle
of karmic dysfunction in the family resulting from reincarnation back into the blood line may be averted or lessened. Forgiveness and acceptance are key here. It is best achieved while
everyone is alive, but in African tradition, forgiveness and healing can occur even when the spirit has passed on. If the trans-
gression from either side is not addressed, the problem may
not only have a harmful effect on the living in this lifetime, but
could continue into the next incarnation in a child or grandchild. Forgiveness is key to healing. Guilt, shame, remorse and

self-condemnation need to be appeased in the spirit world as well. Of course it is better to give forgiveness before a loved one passes over. Sadly, we often wait until it is too late. According to African belief it is never too late, and the spirits can be helped even in the beyond. As children we should take the first step to release our parents and grandparents from blame and then heal past wounds, even if we were the ones to suffer from them. If not, the wound may be carried down through our own progeny. This will occur not only because of the perpetuation of unskilled parenting but also because a troubled spirit may be reborn into the same family, and a similar dysfunction might recur. Pardon will help prevent the same affliction from being passed down from generation to generation.

> *"The most completing gift we can experience is forgiveness,*
> *for we all have its sweet need."*
> John O'Donohue

The Native Americans believe that anything we do will affect the next seven generations. This concurs with the biblical principle that "the sins of the fathers [and mothers] are visited upon the children unto the fourth generation." Fortunately, unhappy, intrusive family spirits that create dysfunction can be released from adverse karmic consequences with rituals embracing forgiveness. The commandment, "Honor your father and mother, that your days will be long upon the earth" is confirmation that the onus is on the child or grandchild to reach out and forgive or ask for forgiveness. The commandment is interesting since it is the only one that states, "... that your days will be long upon the earth." *Sangomas* would explain that this makes sense because that ancestor would then be inclined to help and protect one from the beyond. For those who have suffered greatly at the hands of their parents or grandparents, the commandment instructs us to honor them, not necessarily to love or even like them. Ritual is an effective way to make reparations to the dead. This principle lies at the heart of the *sangoma's* work. All healing eventually comes down to our relationship not only with one's Self but with other living selves, and also with the dead.

Forgiveness is healthful, and the one doing the forgiving benefits even more than the one who is forgiven. Patients with AIDS who have forgiven the person who gave them the virus live much longer and have higher T cell counts than those that have not. Also, there is nothing good about being haunted by an intrusive spirit who is seeking this release. The energy of the spirit gets in the way of the life force of the living being and can cause bad luck, anxiety, depression, trouble with relationships, etc. No matter how difficult it is, there comes a time when one has to be prepared to release those sins perpetrated on oneself, let go, forgive and move on.

Another cannot help you neutralize anything you have not freely, willingly and deliberately given up or want to give up.

One also has to take responsibility for the healing process. Herein lies the power of personal prayer to the Great Spirit and the ancestors, who can mediate on our behalf with or without the help of the *sangoma* or shaman.

The beginning of healing is acknowledging our own pain and where it is and taking tender responsibility for it.

However, one must go beyond being true to oneself and caring for the other. We must let ourselves be cared for by the other. Being willing to be vulnerable is the substance of trust.

No matter how dismal the prognosis, anything can be reversed or improved by the Creator, with or without help from the spirit world, but we have to acknowledge it and want to be free from it. The ancestors are the mediators between us and the Great Spirit and are there to channel Divine healing energy, which is really just love in disguise.

The power of prayer is greater than the power of prophecy [the prognosis], and therein is where healing is to be found. Personal healing is to be found in personal prayer.

We all have permission to go directly to the Great Spirit for help, as well as to our spirit guides.

The *sangoma's* diagnostic repertoire includes trance-possession, bone divination and dream seeing. During spirit possession the ancestral spirit comes "down" from the cosmic "Field" and possesses the healer. The spirit occupies the *sangoma's* body while his or her ego or persona steps aside. In this way healers can access information that is not localized in space and time, since spirits are not confined to the space/time continuum as we are. In this way the *sangoma's* ancestor is able to speak directly to the patient with information highly specific to that individual. We describe this process in the West as "channeling" or "trance-channeling."

THE BONES

The practice of throwing divining bones probably developed over time because healers found spirit mediumship too exhausting. Becoming possessed from drumming and dancing, which can go on all night, is hard work. With this alone it would be impossible to treat very many patients. The bones are another way of allowing the ancestral spirits to have a conversation with the client through the healer.

Reading the bones is a little like unraveling the metaphor of a dream. The healer becomes an interpreter and messenger for the ancestral spirit, who sets up an information field that is accessible to the healer through the bones. When the bones are thrown they do not fall in a random fashion, but in a way that the ancestral spirit controls. A meaningful and usually highly accurate interpretation can then be made by the *sangoma*.

If you were to visit a *sangoma* who, without knowing you, could diagnose your health situation in the past, present, and future, you would be receiving information not localized in time. If at the same time he were to tell you about the health of a loved one living in another country, this would be information not localized in space. These shamans are now called "medical intuitives" in the West. The diagnostic information they can provide can be uncannily accurate. This information has been, and is, available to all peoples in Southern Africa through the *sangomas*, with the help of the ancestral spirits.

Today, few would question the interaction between mind and body, but forty years ago we were still searching for purely mechanical explanations for diseases that were actually rooted in psychological causes. Non-local medicine has yet to become mainstream, but with the help of quantum physics it is now coming into its own. Accessing the "Field" or spirit world and the use of non-local techniques is common not only to traditional or indigenous healers in South Africa, but also to shamans and psychics worldwide. Just as *sangomas* are able to receive non-local information for diagnosis, they are also capable of transmitting distant healing through the medium of their guiding spirits, who become channels for universal healing energy. The healing power that heals the patient is simply Divine love coming from the Great Spirit.

Although most medical doctors today would not agree with the concept of non-local medicine and are still confined by their scientific method and "evidence-based medicine," they would do well to remember Einstein's quote that, "not everything that counts can be counted and not everything that can be counted counts." The ancestors agree in saying that ...

Information is not to be equated with knowledge, knowledge
is not to be equated with understanding, and understanding
is not to be equated with wisdom.

The medical establishment needs to recognize that the scientific method being followed at the moment is more Newtonian than quantum, and hence is somewhat out of date.

There is a protocol for bone divination with any *sangoma* or *nyanga*. The consultation takes place in an *ndumba*, a sacred healing hut where the ancestors are gathered. First, out of respect, you must take off your shoes. The client places a fee under a grass mat, and a rattle is shaken or a chant intoned to call the spirits. Sometimes the healer will make a burnt offering of mpepho, a plant with a pleasant smell that is used similarly to sage used in Native American tradition. The purpose of all these rituals is to open a sacred space into which the spirits are summoned. The healer's bones are contained in a skin or woven grass bag. The healer asks the patient to pick up the bones and put them into the bag and an offering, usually of tobacco, is made. The client shakes the bag of bones, blows into the opening of the bag, states his or her name, and empties the bones onto a mat. The *sangoma* reads the message that has been "thrown" by the spirit guide presiding. Different *sangomas* have differing customs as to how the procedure is conducted, which depend on the idiosyncrasies of their spirit guide.

In my case, I am very fortunate to have a black spirit guide assist in my divinations. She was a *sangoma* in her previous life and hence is very skilled in manipulating the bones and sending the messages and metaphors that I need to translate and convey to my patients. I was told early on in my initiation that, by allowing her to help me, I was also helping her complete the work she had not finished in her previous life. Sometimes spirit guides are able to do karmic work once they are on the other side that they otherwise would not be able to do. Once we die and cross over, usually there is nothing we can do to improve our karma other than reincarnating again – we lose our free will. There is an exception, however, in the case of "enlightened beings," whose free will is retained, which enables them to work without restraints from the beyond.

When dead you can influence on behalf of others but not for yourself. The last chance for determining and acting for your own mission and fulfillment is with your last earthly breath. You are then stuck with how you are and

*where you were until your next incarnation on the long
journey to purify the soul.*

*On the other side of the veil we no longer have options
upon which to decide what fashions our destiny.
We have already determined it.
We do, however, still have thought, intent and opinion
that we may use to help others, though no longer ourselves.
Thus the ancestors need our help just as we need theirs.
Forgiveness, love and gratitude are how we help them.*

Another way the ancestors communicate with the *sangoma* or *nyanga* is through dreams. Interpretation of dreams, as addressed in a previous chapter, is a vital tool of the *sangoma*. Apart from dreaming plant remedies for their patients, other psychic information can be sent through dreams to assist the *sangoma* in caring for the patient.

*Let the dreams guide, and let the bones inform, they each
will help the work of the other.*

MUTI

The medicine, or *muti*, that is used is based on plants and sometimes various animals. This *muti* may have pharmacological properties, but one cannot isolate the power of the remedy from the strength of the healer or that of the ancestors. This phenomenon is another example of the combination of placebo and distant healing. The *muti*s often have powerful symbolism; for instance, lion fat may be used to promote courage. Each time the *muti* is used, it may be accompanied by a ritual which confirms the intention, acts as a powerful affirmation, and allows the spirit guides to help you, with your permission, in that moment remembering that free will is a cosmic law.

In the West, we now know that people can be healed by distant healing or prayer, even if they are unaware they are being healed or prayed for – in other words, placebo is discounted. An increasing number of double-blind studies conducted by Western doctors are showing that distant healing or prayer is statistically significant in improving the outcomes for afflicted patients. These studies usually involve two comparable groups of patients. One group gets standard care, while the other gets standard care plus distant healing or prayer. The latter group has no idea they are receiving healing. In some studies the results are so much better for the group receiving the "non-local therapy" that if the effect could be packaged into a pill, one might be found negligent for omitting it.

The effect of *muti* may be a sophisticated version of distant healing, when the *sangoma's* prayers and ancestors' intentions accompany the treatment. Since the ancestors have access to universal healing energy coming from the Creator, they have the ability to cure almost anything.

Each *muti* carries a different message about what is needed for a particular problem. There is a mutual understanding between healer and ancestor based on tradition, dreams, and empiricism as to what plant to use for various complaints. There are medicines for every eventuality: physical illness, mental illness, social disharmony (such as marital problems), and spiritual difficulties (for instance to align with the ancestors, to get rid of offending spirits, and so on). There are also protective potions and medicines for dreams and luck, among others. In my *sangoma* practice I have focused on *muti*s for psycho-socio-spiritual health. *muti*s, talismans, rituals, chants, drumming and dancing are all containers for blessings.

> *Blessings must have a container, otherwise they cannot be received. One must look to this when one imparts a blessing. The container can be a stone, a song, a plant, a prayer, a chant, a bit of bread, a sip of wine or a mystical incantation. Because of their function containers are blessings in themselves and they themselves have the power to bless.*

CAUSES OF ILLNESS

There are three main causes of illness: spiritual intrusions, witchcraft or sorcery, and ritual impurity or pollution. Illness can also just be physical and have no clear explanation, or it may come directly from God. Even benevolent ancestors may indirectly cause illness by turning away from their progeny. The ancestor, or calling, or *Thwasa* sickness has been addressed in the text. If the ancestors feel they are being ignored, they may cause harm by omission rather than commission. In feeling neglected, they may abandon their loved ones and no longer afford them protection. Sometimes an ancestor may want a loved one to join him on the other side; this can also result in sickness. Malevolent ancestors, and particularly vindictive foreign spirits who may or may not have been wronged, can also cause illness, misfortune, accidents, and death, even for the descendants of those who have wronged them. These maladies can be counteracted by prayers, rituals, *muti* and sacrifices. Ancestors who have turned away can be encouraged to return and defend against malicious or intruding spirits. Illness is therefore frequently connected to human relationships between the living and the dead. If these relationships are perfectly functional and healthy, the *sangoma* will look to witchcraft, sorcery or pollution for the cause of the problem.

Pollution, which might better be called ritual impurity, occurs as a result of contact with some occurrence or phenomenon that is impure. Causes of pollution include miscarriages, birth, illness, crime, death (especially murder), menses, pregnancy, sex, a journey, meat of an animal that died of disease, and pork. Many *sangomas* will purify themselves after sex and after attending funerals or corpses. A spouse is polluted for a period of time after the death of a wife, husband or child.

While a healer can heal someone far away, a sorcerer can create disease and even death from a distance with a hex. White or black magic has been known for millennia, but is only now being validated by science. Although it sounds implausible to the Western mind, in South Africa, traditional healers deal with witchcraft every day. These malevolent effects can be local or non-local. Non-local influences work through the Field without the knowledge of those who are affected. Local effects work directly on the inner healer with the knowledge of the victim through the nocebo effect.

The key to nocebo and placebo is the belief system of the patient, the absence or presence of hope, belief, trust, and faith. We are all aware of the doctor-patient relationship and how important it is for healing. Just as some physicians create a feeling of calm, confidence, and reassurance in their patients, others can do the opposite. Some doctors will engender the healing power of placebo, others the noxiousness of nocebo. Placebo is about love and nocebo about fear.

When using words you should choose them well. Never use them as a weapon to harm or as an alienating defense but rather for explanation and instruction and sometimes to clearly dissuade, support, release, encourage, alert and reassure.

If you perceive uncertainly or a need, let the words simply acknowledge and nourish.

If they do not inform, inspire, give comfort or bring laughter do not use them.

Distant healing, or its opposite, the hex, work through the Field, bypassing the belief system of the recipient. The Field, like our inner healer (and the Internet), is not impervious to bad morals or evil motivation. Witchcraft and sorcery are very much part of the *Tshisimane* saga and are related in that chapter in the text. P.H. said to me early on during my *Thwasa* that there was always a temptation to go over to the dark side for financial gain, since doing so could be extremely lucrative.

There are various grades of severity when it comes to witchcraft, but in essence, anything that interferes with another's free will could be considered witchcraft. Hence a love potion to solicit sexual favors from someone is odious, and quite different from giving someone a strengthening potion so that they can present themselves to a prospective partner in the most optimal way. Working spells to cause one's business competition to be less successful, or an opposing soccer team to play poorly, are also not in line with the intentions of guiding spirits that work in the light.

Many healers have forgotten the source of their and the
ancestors' power. Their empowerment to help others, and
realize and use their own empowerment,
has been weakened. Even with good intentions, many are
falling into superstition. If one is not aware, humble and
grateful it is easy to mislead and misuse.

Africans believe that the dead are not dead and that our ancestors are there to help, protect and sustain us. They cannot communicate with us in the normal way since they live in the realm of spirit, but they are there nonetheless. Many of us never even knew our grandparents, and certainly pay no tribute either to them or to parents long gone. Those of us who have had inattentive children know how easy it is to turn away from even a loved child when a relationship is not nourished. The same is true for ancestors. As P.H. often repeated, "If your ancestors turn aside, you are defenseless in life, like papers blowing in the wind." He also taught that we "lift up" our ancestors by revering and remembering them – *"pagamisa"* in Zulu.

It's an interesting reversal that as more and more blacks in South Africa are drawn to a Western way of life, more and more whites are seeking out the wisdom of ancient Africa. There are more than 250,000 *sangomas* in South Africa, and an ever-increasing number of white ones, too. *Sangomas* are still ubiquitous in South Africa, and they continue to play a pivotal role in the health and wholeness of the post-apartheid new South Africa.

David cumes, md

The results of healing may not manifest in a way seen by
seeing eyes, nor in time as kept by clock and calendar.
It will unfold in its season, which will sometimes be as a
sudden cloudburst and at others as a butterfly emerging
and at still others as a harvest long after the planting.
Each will be according to the nature of the healing needs
of the patient.

APPENDIX 2

searching for universals: sangomas and the Lemba

Those who exploit knowledge are lost to wisdom. Wisdom is born of humility and is nourished by compassion. It is grace in action. When knowledge is used for only self-gain and control it is conceit in action.

VENDA HAS BEEN CALLED THE LAND OF LEGEND, THE LAND of mists and myths. Rider Haggard wrote about it in his novel, King Solomon's Mines, that I had read as a boy. I realized that it was no accident that my dreams had pointed me to *Tshisimane*. I had been enchanted by the magic of the descriptions of the land many years ago.

While I was doing my initiation, I was struck by the "Old Testament-like" nature of much of the information I was receiving, and the rituals I participated in often felt very biblical. Two years later, when I arrived in Limpopo and became more familiar with the culture, I learned about the Lemba people.

There is a tribe, called the Balemba or the Lemba (in Venda), that are unique in that they have always claimed that they were black Jews. Recently, genetic studies have proved them correct. In fact many in the Buba clan were found to be Kohanim or members of the priestly sect of the Israelites, possibly dating back to Aaron, Moses' brother, and possibly even to the patriarch Jacob. Other Lemba tribes have Hebrew-like names.

The Lemba adhere to many distinctly Jewish customs. Traditionally they did not intermarry, but this has changed. They circumcise the boys at the age of eight years (rather than eight days), slaughter their animals in a kosher fashion, and do not eat pork. They bury their dead facing north and in a horizontal rather than a sitting position, as do the Venda people. Their emblem is an elephant inside the Star of David and this adorns their graves. They also have distinctly Jewish laws in relation to ritual purity, and some of the people look Semitic.

Women are considered ritually impure during menstruation, as are medicine men or women who attend a corpse. Anyone who eats road kill or an animal that has died of natural causes is also impure. This ritual impurity requires cleansing, and women undergo ritual purification after menstruating or giving birth. All of these concepts can be found in the Old Testament, and it seemed clear to me that many other Bantu peoples had also been practicing some of these laws long before being introduced to the Bible by the missionaries. Neither were any of these practices found in the Christian faith.

It is hard to know fact from legend, but the Lemba believe that they are descendants of Solomon. Possibly after Nebuchadnezzar sacked the temple, around 700 B.C., they may have migrated south instead of being forced to go into exile in Babylon. Alternatively, when the Israelites were released from exile in Babylon and allowed to return home, some may have migrated south instead. There are many theories as to their origins. They seem to have first journeyed to Yemen, to a place called Senna, where they lived for some time. They then crossed the Indian Ocean and trekked down the eastern side of Africa. Some migrated across the Limpopo River into what is now called Venda, while the rest remained in Zimbabwe. Still others earlier on might have gone west to Ethiopia to become the Falashas.

The Lemba were also warriors with expertise in making metal weapons. The Great God, Mwari, gave them a sacred drum or Ngoma Lugundu, the drum that thunders. Before engaging in battle with tribes they encountered, they would sound the drum, which apparently made them invincible. The drum was carried on poles, much like the Hebrew Ark of the Covenant, and was never to touch the ground. They were also duty-bound to keep to their traditions, but when they arrived at the Limpopo River, it seems they intermarried and became lax with their laws. The sacred drum fell on the ground, and after that misfortune overtook them.

Recently a 600-year-old drum resembling the *Ngoma Lugundu* was rediscovered in the Harare museum by the Lemba scholar Tudor Parfitt. The drum has features which look Hebraic, but it had been severely burnt. It was constructed so that it could be carried on poles, but it is believed not to be the original drum.

The Lemba are a paradoxical population of tens of thousands of self-proclaimed Jews who live mostly in Malawi, Zimbabwe and in Venda, and their true history is shrouded in legend. Many who today follow Christianity or Islam still proudly lay claim to their Jewish heritage. Old maps of the Holy Land have revealed that there was a place called Lemba long ago, before the Christian era. There are about 70,000 Lemba in Southern Africa.

If one looks at the spirituality of Southern African tribes, especially in the north, one recognizes a distinct biblical ethos. It is also true that one can discover these universal truths among many indigenous peoples wherever they are. The reason for this may be that truth, like cream, always "rises to the top." Nevertheless, during my initiation and later studies, I could not fail to notice how many of the principles of Bantu spirituality can also be found in the Old Testament. The Lemba may have brought the ritual of circumcision to Venda, and from there it may have spread further south. Many non-Lemba *sangomas* also do not eat pork, although wild pig bones are represented in most divination bone sets. The Lemba, however, have no history of having a Torah. Other Southern African tribes had no Bible, Koran, Vedas or sacred texts to learn from. Neither did they have any writing; theirs was an oral tradition.

I was puzzled as to why it is that the Bantu peoples, and the Bushmen of Southern Africa, had such sophisticated psycho-spiritual abilities, when we in the West, with all our education, seem to be lacking in these dimensions. An explanation for the advanced spiritual skills of Africa's indigenous peoples may lie in the fact that they have been living in close proximity to nature and the earth: the Garden of Eden archetype.

Rabbi Yochanan, a famous Kabbalist, wrote: *"If we did not have the Torah we could have learned it from the animals."*

I believe that the Bushmen hunter-gatherers in particular, and also their more agrarian Bantu neighbors, learned similar spiritual and healing secrets from their contact with nature, coupled with being able to stay close to their primal intelligence and natural rhythms. We have paid a price for our modern technology, and our left-brain oriented education has separated us from nature's wisdom and its primeval energies. Sadly, the pure indigenous knowledge, that has until recently only been taught by word of mouth, is now slowly being polluted by adoption of our modern way of life.

"Nature hides her secrets with consummate modesty and speaks usually in an unintelligible tongue."
Charles Huggins

Within nature lies the secret tongue of the Great Spirit, or what Kabbalah would call the Sod – the secret. The Bushmen and the Bantu have studied and mastered the essence of this language. When I began my initiation process in Swaziland in 2000, P.H. Mntshali said to me, "This is the original medicine; it will never change – just like the law of gravity." In the West we are victims of our religions, education, culture, and conditioning. We are unable to fathom how disconnected we are from our original humanness. We need to recognize how much we have forfeited and how much we can learn from native peoples who can access these spiritual realms with such ease. We all need liberal amounts of time reconnecting with our Earth Mother. We also need to protect and sustain her. African wisdom has the extraordinary ability to "see" across the veil between worlds. A good friend of mine, Izak Barnard, who had spent most of his life learning from the Bushmen, once said to me, "Dave, we may be the masters of technology, but the Bushmen and the Bantu are the masters of the spiritual world."

It was apparent to us that part of the ancestral "contract" with Maryellen and me was to try to revive some of the ancient

Hebrew shamanic knowledge and show parallels with its African relative. This was one example:

"Vulture came down and the dead animals were restored.
Vulture brings vision and rebirth, redeems and purifies.
Vulture is a carrier of the breath of life."

Also in a dream, an old patriarch appeared with Maryellen and me, along with a vulture, saying, *"You are as you do, not as you appear. Regard the golden purifier!"* I asked the vulture if he would teach me to see beyond my sight. He looked at me as if deciding something and then touched me with his wings, and I floated upwards.

Early on in my association with Maryellen, James, a deceased Lemba, appeared as a spirit guide. He was tall, well built, handsome, bald and usually dressed in resplendent clothing or a white tunic. He visited us from time to time with messages of encouragement. On one occasion the visit was associated with the symbol of the Lemba, the elephant inside the Star of David.

Ancient Hebrew shamans believed in the powers inherent in different animals – for instance, the eagle was an animal of compassion, the vulture was endowed with insight, and the raven was known to be the trickster. In *sangoma* medicine vulture *muti* is used to facilitate one's ability to "see" and divine.

Kabbalists describe a *Veil of Illusion* that must be bridged in order to talk to their teachers on the other side. *Sangomas* and Bushman shamans are also experts in crossing this veil.

In the divination set of the *sangoma*, each animal is endowed with its own unique essence. For instance, the anteater is the animal that digs the grave, and this bone talks of death or spirits on the other side. Hence, when the bones are thrown, the anteater bone, which is manipulated by the energy field of the spirit guide, knows exactly where to fall and in what orientation to lie. According to Jewish thinking it is believed that each of us is endowed with a special bone in the spine that gives us our unique essence, or Etzem. Bones appear to have immense spiritual power. Elephants have been seen doing rituals with the bones of their departed ones. They visit them and even use them in a type of funeral procession in which they will walk in a line and respectfully hand a bone of the dead elephant back along the line with their trunks.

Sangomas can use divination to diagnose clients who have *"shades"* that are hanging around trying to get the attention of their progeny so they can be forgiven and released from the misdeeds of the past. When I first studied the bones I was introduced to the concept of *"shade,"* which is an intrusive spirit or entity that is bothering the living. I found out after my initiation that the word *"sheyd,"* plural *"sheydim,"* is actually a Hebrew word found in Kabbalah and applies to a ghost or similar entity. Possibly this word was introduced by the Lemba long ago. Rituals, often involving animal sacrifice, are performed to release shades. Furthermore, if the *"shade"* or ghost of the ancestor is forgiven and released, he or she can get on with a more optimistic karmic future. Just as animal sacrifice was practiced in Temple days by the Hebrews as the ultimate atonement for sins against God, so for *sangomas*, animal sacrifice is the ultimate restitution that is made to an ancestor concerning guilt, shame and remorse.

Sangomas recognize another condition that can cause "dis-ease," and eventually disease, apart from intrusive spirits. It is called pollution or something that is "dirty" by the Zulus, but is better labeled as ritual impurity. One can find reference to many of these same ritual impurities in Leviticus. In biblical times, anyone who had been in contact with a dead body, or who had eaten a dead animal that had not been killed in a Kosher manner, was not allowed back into the community until he or she had been purified. Religious Jewish women are not allowed to be in contact with their husbands during menstruation. They are also required to have a ritual bath before having sexual intercourse with their husbands after menstruation has ended.

Sangomas also recognize a state of ritual impurity resulting from sex during menses, contact with a corpse, and eating a dead animal found in the bush or road kill. African thinking believes that a woman is very powerful on her "moon" cycle, and that this force can overwhelm a man who has sex with her and make him sick. The concept is really a tribute to the unique power of feminine energy rather than an issue of "pollution," which could be considered offensive in nature.

Red is a protective, cleansing color not only among Kabbalists but also in *sangoma* medicine. Plants used for ritual purification because of sex during menses are frequently red in color. Purification in the Old Testament was done with ashes from a red heifer and the red dye of a particular worm.

Attending a corpse is a meritorious service, but still carries the implications of ritual impurity or energetic pollution that needs to be corrected for balance. Several times I have visited a *sangoma* only to find that he was officiating at a funeral. When I would say that I would wait until he was finished I was invariably told to come back the next day, since the *sangoma* would not do any work until after he had purified himself. On one occasion I witnessed a Bushman shaman exorcising the polluting energy of a puff adder from a woman who had cooked and eaten the deadly snake a week previously. I once needed to have the spirit or energy of a dog I had to put down because it was suffering exorcised by *Femba*. The spirit of the dog had attached itself to me while being euthanized. The *sangoma* who did the ritual knew nothing of the fact that I had done this three weeks previously, 300 miles away.

Pollution can occur after a journey, and objects may also be ritually impure, as in the case of the story of the ceramic pots that Rupert sequestered from a cave.

There are recommendations in the Bible about impurity and the idea that even land or a place can be severely polluted or cursed. Sometimes fire is the only thing that can purify demonic evil and malevolence.

You shall tear down their altars and smash their sacred pillars and burn their Asherim with fire, and you shall cut down the engraved images of their gods and obliterate their name from that place. (Deuteronomy 12:3)

Or, as stated by the ancestors:

Demonic worship is often practiced with such zealotry, determination and passion that its power has a lasting force for captivating and destroying. It is best that one not try to remove the rotten and decaying apples from the pile, but rather move the good apples far away. In some instances, if the stench and rot still present danger, then it may be appropriate for a cleansing, sterilizing and purifying to take place, but only by knowledgeable specialists in such matters.

During George's initiation as a *sangoma*, his training included the spiritual clearing out and cleansing of homesteads, businesses and even objects. This can be dangerous work, especially if there are evil spirits present. African belief is that fire can destroy or evict malevolent spirits. An Inward Bound group member that I once took to see a skilled *sangoma* in Venda was alarmed when she was told that her house was occupied by a malevolent spirit and that she should burn it down and move somewhere else. Usually *sangomas* do not have to resort to such drastic methods and cleansing can be done with *mutis*, rituals and with the help of the ancestors. *Sangomas* have rituals and medicines for all of these "biblical" pathologies, including rituals for funerals, bereavement and especially, in the case of the Zulu, a warrior people, for purification after war.

As quoted in Job, *"God's purpose in so treating man is to lead him to himself and away from the pit."* (Job 33:17) It seems that African spirituality was also well aware of the subtle energies that can lead humans to the "pit." The Lemba may have contributed to some of these understandings, but they had no Torah, although they may have carried with them some of the oral equivalent. Many of these principles can also be found among other indigenous peoples on different continents. They are best called universal truths, but our modern way of life has discarded this wisdom as primitive, superstitious thinking.

God's cosmic law is free will, and African understandings are well aware of this. It is implicit in the divinatory process and in dream interpretation. The bones and the dreams tell you "what to see, not what to be!" What you do with the information is up to you. Hence the ancestors explain:

the source

The results of cause and effect (or karma) are often not immediate because it would influence free will. God wants us to do things for the right reasons, not out of fear and shame and because of what may result, but out of love and justice.

Free will, as we tend to think of it, implies choices so that we may decide upon them. Where there are no choices there is no freedom of will to be exercised. Where choices are limited by circumstances, one may still at least determine what one's attitude will be and how to respond, not in action, but in deciding thought, intent and opinion.

There is no free will across the veil except in the enlightenment realms. The dead depend on the living to repair, complete, forgive and release them if such is needed.

Reincarnation is inevitable for those of us who are not Self-realized on our long journeys to purify our souls so that we can attain perfection. We can, however, improve our karma and the potential for spiritual progress in our next life by doing service from the other side of the veil. This requires the permission of the living because of free will. My ancestor who helps me with bone divination is completing, through me, work she did not accomplish in her previous incarnation as a *sangoma*. By allowing her to help me I "lift her up" (*pagamisa* in Zulu). She in return helps me immeasurably.

African thinking, like Kabbalah and other ancient wisdom traditions, embraces the idea of paradox. They, too, recognize that light and dark must coexist; there cannot be one without the other. However, since none of these concepts have been written down until recently, one has had to sit at the feet of a master *sangoma* who may not even be able to read or write to slowly glean them.

Since we all arose in Africa, the origins of all healing can be found there. Western science is now discovering, with the non-locality of quantum theory, many "new" principles which *sangomas* have known for eons. We are now going back to what we once knew.

GLOSSARY

Bakkie (Afrikaans) – pickup truck
Boerewors (Afrikaans) – "farmer's" sausage, usually made with beef and pork
Braai (Afrikaans) – barbecue
Budlu (Zulu) – a herbal brew

Curandero (Spanish) – shaman

Etzem (Hebrew) – a bone in the spine that gives each individual his or her unique essence

Femba (Zulu) – a form of psycho-spiritual diagnosis and cleansing or exorcism done in a state of trance possession
"Field" – the knowable and unknowable world of spirit

Hammerkop (Afrikaans) – "hammer head" – a powerful mystical bird used by witches to cause harm; sometimes called the lightning bird

Impundulu (Zulu) – a *Hammerkop*
Inyanga (Zulu) – a traditional healer who relies more on divination and dreams than on trance for diagnosis (*Nyanga* in Zimbabwe)

Kabbalah (Hebrew) – the Jewish mystical belief
Kahuna (Hawaiian) - – shaman in Hawaii
Kia (Kung Bushmen) – out of body spirit flight
Kiepersol (Afrikaans) – cabbage tree, Cussonia species
Kohanim (Hebrew) – the priestly sect of the Israelites
Kraal (Afrikaans) – a cattle enclosure
Kunda (Hindu) from the word *Kundalini* – something that is coiled; can also mean a pool

Kundalini (Hindu) – the feminine serpent power that rests at the coccyx that can ascend up the central energetic channel of the spine and is key to spiritual transformation and transcendence

Lapa (Afrikaans) – a covered outdoor area used for *braaing* and entertaining
Lemba or **Balemba** – the black Jews of Southern Africa who reside in the northern regions including Zimbabwe

Maggidim (Hebrew) – discarnate Jewish sages
Malpitte (Afrikaans) – "seeds that make you mad" from the Datura plant
Mampoor (Afrikaans) – moonshine
Mandawe or **Ummandawu** (Zulu) – a powerful indigenous African spirit
Mfesi (Zulu) – Mozambique spitting cobra
Middelmannetjie (Afrikaans) – the raised ridge in the middle of a dirt road created by off-road travel
Modimo (Sotho) – God
Moya (Zulu) – spirit
Mpepho (Zulu) – a plant burned to attract the attention of the ancestors
Muti (Zulu) – traditional African medicine
Mwari (Lemba) – God

Ndumba (Zulu) – healing hut where the ancestors reside and help heal, classically round with adobe walls and a thatched roof
Ngoma (Zulu) – drum (also the derivation of the word *sangoma*)
Ngoma lugundu (Lemba) – the drum that thunders
Num (Kung Bushmen) – equivalent of the yoga *Kundalini*

Oran Mor (Celtic) – the music that fills all creation with its Divine harmony

Pagamisa (Zulu) – to "lift up" or honor the ancestors

Pargawd (Hebrew) – the veil between our world of matter and the world of God and spirit

Ruach (Hebrew) – literally means wind, but can refer to spirit

Sangoma (Zulu) – a traditional healer in South Africa
Sanusi (Zulu) – a high Zulu prophet
Shade – an intrusive spirit (possibly from the Hebrew word **Sheyd** with the same meaning)
Siswati – the language of the Swazi people
Skelm (Afrikaans) – a trickster
Soutpansberg (Afrikaans) – Salt Pan Mountains; a mountain range in the far north of South Africa, close to the Limpopo River

Thwasa (Zulu) – the process of initiation to become a *sangoma*
Tilo (Shangaan) – lightning
Torah (Hebrew) – the Five Books of Moses (the first five books in the Old Testament)
Tshisimane (Venda) – the source, a spring, the Creator, God
Tsotsi (Zulu) – a gangster
Tzaddikim (Hebrew) – righteous or enlightened sages

Umbilini (Zulu) – the place of two; the mystical place in the body where the body and soul unite and become one powerful thing
Umhagate shells (Zulu) – Mangete nut shells used for divination. Also called mongongo or manketti nut or nongongo; nuts from the Schinziophyton rautanenii tree
Umkulunkulu (Zulu) – God
Umthakati (Zulu) – a malevolent witch
Unzunzu (Zulu) – the water spirit

Veldskoen (Afrikaans) – literally a veld shoe; hardy footwear for outdoor use

CPSIA information can be obtained
at www.ICGtesting.com
Printed in the USA
FSOW02n1227261117
41400FS